Secondary Spread
of Cancer

Secondary Spread
of Cancer

Edited by
R. W. BALDWIN
The University of Nottingham
Cancer Research Campaign Laboratories
Nottingham, England

1978

ACADEMIC PRESS
London · New York · San Francisco
A Subsidiary of Harcourt Brace Jovanovich, Publishers

ACADEMIC PRESS INC. (LONDON) LTD
24/28 Oval Road
London NW1

United States Edition published by
ACADEMIC PRESS INC.
111 Fifth Avenue
New York, New York 10003

Library of Congress Catalog Card Number: 77-79299
ISBN: 0-12-076850-X

Printed in Great Britain by
William Clowes & Sons Limited
London, Beccles and Colchester

List of Contributors

R. W. BALDWIN, *The University of Nottingham, Cancer Research Campaign Laboratories, University Park, Nottingham, England*

R. L. CARTER, *Institute of Cancer Research, Royal Cancer Hospital, The Haddow Laboratories, Clifton Avenue, Sutton, Surrey, England*

STEPHEN K. CARTER, *Northern California Cancer Program, 1801 Page Mill Road, Bldg B/Suite 200, Palo Alto, California 94304, USA*

SILVIO GARATTINI, *Istituto di Ricerche Farmacologiche "Mario Negri", Via Eritrea 62, 20157 Milano, Italy*

L. N. OWEN, *Department of Veterinary Clinical Medicine, School of Veterinary Medicine, Cambridge, England*

M. V. PIMM, *The University of Nottingham, Cancer Research Campaign Laboratories, University Park, Nottingham, England*

FREDERICO SPREAFICO, *Istituto di Ricerche Farmacologiche "Mario Negri", Via Eritrea 62, 20157 Milano, Italy*

J. STJERNSWÄRD, *Ludwig Institute for Cancer Research (Lausanne Branch) and Department of Radiotherapy, Cantonal University Hospital, Lausanne, Switzerland*

C. F. VON ESSEN, *Swiss Institute of Nuclear Research, 5234 Villigen, Switzerland*

Preface

The single most important characteristic of malignant cells is their capacity to metastasise, so producing tumours at distant sites. Indeed were it not for this property, many more patients could be cured by treatment of the primary growth. It is at first sight surprising therefore to find how little attention has been given until quite recently to the study of the processes of cancer cell dissemination. A closer examination of the problem indicates, however, how complex are these metastatic processes and their study is limited by the still rather rudimentary understanding of the control mechanisms involved in the growth of malignant cells. The primary objective of this book, therefore, is to present short authoritative accounts of several approaches for studying metastasis, and the treatment of secondary tumour growths. It will be immediately apparent to the reader how limited are the developments in many of these approaches under review and hopefully the challenge will be taken up by future research. One challenge for the experimentalist is to explain why with many animal tumours, such as those induced by extrinsic agents, e.g. chemical carcinogens, metastatic spread is not as common a feature as in clinical cancer. Does this mean that many of the experimental animal tumours lack an important property as analogues of human cancer, and, as reviewed in Chapter V, should other animal species be considered? Indeed, it would be a worthwhile study to compare the physio-pathological properties of tumours developing in one species with different metastatic potentials (Chapter I). This would surely include a closer look at the cell surface and particularly the accumulation (binding) of macro-molecules such as proteases, since many feel that the release of tumour cells from a primary tumour is controlled primarily by cell–cell interactions. Undoubtedly the tumour immunologist has much to offer in this type of investigation, although at present little effort has been made to turn loose the sophisticated immunological technology for characterizing metastasising and non-metastasising tumour cells (Chapter VI). Equally, these procedures will find use for studying what might be the more important question of how a disseminated tumour cell finds a "home" in which it is able to lie dormant, often for considerable periods of time, until an as yet undefined signal or set of signals induces this cell to proliferate progressively to become a metastatic growth (Chapter II).

Included in the book are a number of accounts of possible approaches to the treatment of metastatic disease. These include a consideration of the role of chemotherapy (Chapters IV and VII) where the point is made that too little attention has yet been given to agents which may influence the process of tumour cell dissemination (Chapter IV). It is perhaps necessary to work on the assumption that clinically when a primary tumour is treated, at least occult metastases are already present which also require treatment. The role of radiotherapy is considered in this respect (Chapter III) and the controversial view that radiation of tissues may under certain circumstances enhance metastatic disease requires challenge. The reader should also be cautioned about accepting too readily the view that immunotherapy holds out a ready and simple method for treating metastatic disease (Chapter VI). Nothing in tumour immunology is simple, and the principles of immunotherapy are still ill-defined. In fact there is to date little animal data to support the view that immunology is effective in treating metastatic deposits, apart from approaches aimed at depositing "macrophage-stimulating" agents such as bacillus Calmette Guérin (BCG) into lesions, and many of the clinical trials remain unproven.

The underlying message of the book is for a more basic and fundamental approach to the study of the processes involved in the release of tumour cells from a primary tumour, and for their subsequent deposition and development in secondary deposits. If as a result of our endeavours, investigators can be encouraged to study this multitude of questions, so providing a firmer basis for clinical studies, the book will have achieved its objective.

December 1977   R. W. B.

Contents

Chapter I

General Pathology of the Metastatic Process

R. L. CARTER

Institute of Cancer Research and Royal Marsden Hospital, Sutton, Surrey, England

> "The peculiarity of cancer lies in its ability to create fresh starting points for a malignant mass when arrested somewhere along the system".
>
> THOMAS HODGKIN (1848)

1. Introduction

The capacity for metastatic spread can reasonably be regarded as the single most important characteristic of malignant tumours. It is also the least understood. The overall march of events which characterize metastasis is easy enough to reconstruct, and competent analyses of some features of the metastatic process were made by writers at the turn of the century (for review, *see* Wilder, 1956; Willis, 1973). But it will soon be apparent from the present chapter that purely descriptive accounts of certain critical phases of metastasis are still lacking and that investigations into underlying mechanisms have barely begun. Detection and treatment of metastatic disease in man continues to pose formidable problems; but slow improvements are being made and the older attitudes of therapeutic nihilism can, in several contexts, be legitimately questioned. It is therefore essential that clinical and experimental investigation into the general

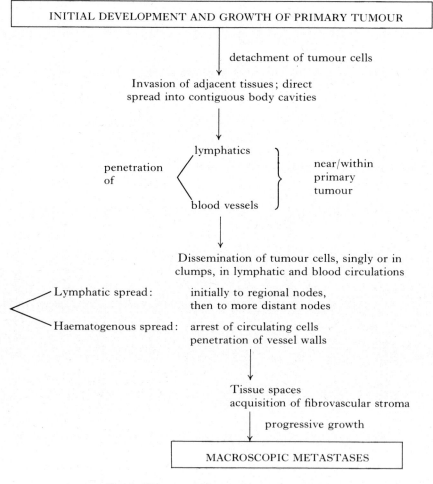

Fig. 1. The natural history of metastatic growth

pathology—or perhaps what might be called the natural history—of the metastatic process is aggressively pursued.

It is convenient to regard metastasis as a series of events each of which can be analysed separately (Fig. 1). It is self-evident that each phase involves a measure of interaction between tumour cells and host elements of various kinds, and it is important to note that the host elements which respond to metastasising tumour involve far more than the immune system, preoccupation with which has tended to obscure the role of stromal reactions, coagulation mechanisms and probably inflammatory responses.

II. The Primary Tumour

Appraisal of the likely metastatic potential of a primary tumour is still little short of rudimentary. In addition to purely clinical aspects, some clues will be afforded to the pathologist by the anatomical site of the tumour and cell of origin, its size, extent of local spread and—in particular— its histological appearances. With most tumours, it is reasonable to link increasing risk of metastasis with decreasing morphological differentiation as judged by conventional light microscopy. Such an association is empirical and based largely on accumulated experience. Specific morphological features are sometimes singled out and used for grading schemes which, in certain tumours, may give more precise prognostic information. Histological signs of local lymphatic or blood vessel invasion by tumour usually provide a clear indication that the metastatic process is already in train. It is, however, well recognized that there are several tumours where microscopy is no guide to metastatic behaviour: the most notable examples occur among cancers of the thyroid, adrenal and ovary. Here, seemingly well-differentiated lesions may metastasise but—paradoxically—histological evidence of local vascular involvement does not necessarily indicate that metastasis has occurred. Again, some malignant neoplasms, irrespective of their degree of morphological differentiation, invade locally but rarely metastasise to distant sites: examples include basal cell tumours, gliomas and thymomas. Exceptionally, embryonal tumours may show morphological signs of maturation with a corresponding improvement in prognosis and decreased risk of spread. The best documented examples are neuroblastomas, some teratomas and retinoblastomas and various other childhood malignancies (Smithers, 1969). The mechanisms for this excessively rare event are unknown.

The presence of host cell infiltrates of lymphocytes, plasma cells and macrophages in and around certain primary tumours— medullary carcinoma of the breast, malignant melanoma, choriocarcinoma, seminoma—is commonly regarded as a favourable prognostic feature; but the relevance of such infiltrates vis-à-vis local invasion and metastasis is unclear. This topic is discussed further in *Chapter II*.

Non-morphological criteria for assessing malignant potential are largely speculative at the present time.

(1) Loss of ABH isoantigens was described by Davidsohn and his co-workers (*see* Davidsohn, 1972) in human primary tumours arising in several different sites: oral cavity, stomach, large intestine, cervix, lung, pancreas, bladder and ovary. Some interesting initial findings were reported, but a recent paper from Davidsohn's group (Lill *et al.*, 1976) casts considerable doubts on the results previously obtained in intraepithelial carcinomas of the cervix. Loss of ABH isoantigens must, therefore, now be viewed with reserve.

(2) Expression of new antigens is a still more problematic determinant of metastatic behaviour. Synthesis and release of previously-suppressed fetal antigens, typified by carcino-embryonic antigen (CEA), may perhaps reflect some tumours' innate metastatic potential as well as serving as a means of monitoring the overall tumour burden. The role of true tumour-specific transplantation antigens in metastatic growth is equally speculative (*see* Chapter VI), though an association between a scanty glycocalyx, low immunogenicity and a high capacity to metastasise has been described in mammary tumours in rats (Kim, 1970; Kim *et al.*, 1975). Corroboration in other experimental tumour systems is needed before human implications can reasonably be considered.

(3) The elaboration and release of certain tumour-associated products may be an important determinant of metastatic behaviour. Examples include factors which stimulate local vasoproliferation or which dissolve bone, both of which are discussed later in this chapter.

It is reasonable to postulate, though difficult to prove, that the neoplastic cells which comprise a tumour are functionally heterogeneous and that certain elements in such a mixed population of malignant cells will have a particular proclivity to metastasise. This problem has been investigated by Fidler (1973a, 1975, 1976) in studies which have produced persuasive evidence that sub-populations of cells with enhanced metastatic potential can be demonstrated within tumours. Using the B16 melanoma which had been adjusted to grow in tissue culture as well as *in vivo*, Fidler (1973a) set up the following system. B16 cells were grown for a short period *in vitro* and then injected intravenously into syngeneic (C57B1) mice where they gave rise to pulmonary deposits. Cells from these deposits were grown up again *in vitro* and injected into normal mice, and the cycle was repeated several times. The incidence of lung tumours increased with each tumour line derived from successive pulmonary metastases. These results suggest the operation of intrinsic properties of the individual tumour cell lines rather than any extraneous factors: and attempts have been made to characterize high- and low-metastasising B16 cell lines in more detail. Fidler (1975) found that the high-metastasis lines showed more invasive ness in the subcutaneous tissues, more trapping in the lungs, more pulmonary metastases and a greater tendency to form clumps with platelets. Bosmann *et al.* (1973) have reported comparative chemical and biophysical investigations with the two lines and, in sparse cultures, these authors found differences in electrophoretic mobility and—significantly—in surface glycoprotein, glycosyltransferases, glycosidases, transferases and proteases. Recently, Winkelhake and Nicolson (1976) have compared the *in vitro* adhesive properties of Fidler's high- and low-metastasising B16 cell lines. They find that the high metastasising lines have a relatively greater capacity to attach to homotypic or heterotypic monolayers—in this case, monolayers of the same B16 cells or 3T3 cells. Subsequent studies with other target organs have proved particularly interesting (Nicolson *et al.*, 1976): the high metastasising B16 lines adhered rapidly and strongly to lung cells but interacted weakly with liver, spleen, heart and other cells. The low metastasising B16 line adhered slowly to all heterotypic cell substrates, showing no target specificity.

A. *Stroma*

The supporting fibrovascular stroma plays an essential role in establishing and maintaining a growing primary tumour and in facilitating its local and distant spread. It has, indeed, been suggested that the rate of proliferation of vascular endothelium is an important factor in limiting the rate of tumour growth (Tannock, 1970)—a proposal that applies equally to primary and metastatic lesions (cf. Section VI). The kinetic turnover of unstimulated capillary endothelium is normally measured in months; endothelium in a transplantable rat mammary adenocarcinoma has a turnover time of about 50 hr, comparable to that found in proliferating endothelium in the vicinity of a 3-day old fracture (Tannock, 1970; Tannock and Hayashi, 1972).

The stimuli which induce endothelial proliferation are likely to be diverse, but one important element is released by the tumour itself—

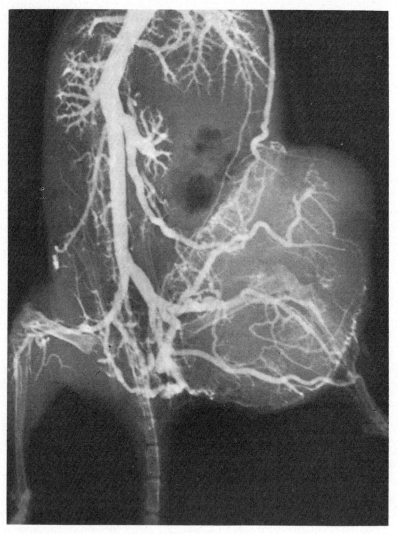

FIG. 2. Venogram of a Lewis carcinoma (3LL) in a C57B1 mouse, 21 days after implantation. Highly vascular zones containing tortuous blood vessels alternate with regions with little or no demonstrable blood supply. (Illustration kindly supplied by Dr. Anne Atherton and Professor K. Hellmann)

the *tumour angiogenesis factor* (TAF) of Folkman (*see* Folkman, 1974, 1975). A reciprocal interaction is thus established between tumour cells and capillary endothelium, aptly described by Folkman as "a highly integrated ecosystem".

Many tumours are richly vascular (Fig. 2) but the detailed anatomy of their blood vessels is still imperfectly understood. Thiersch, in 1865, commented on the abundant growth of capillaries in the stroma of carcinomas, and the current view (*see* Willis, 1973) suggests that most tumour vessels consist only of "irregular endothelium-lined channels with scanty perivascular connective tissue". Investigations with experimental tumours confirm this view (Underwood and Carr, 1972; Papadimitriou and Woods, 1975) and interesting serial studies on vascular morphology and blood flow in developing and regressing Walker tumours in rats have been reported by Oikawa *et al.* (1975).

Blood vessels in experimental tumours have been shown to be highly permeable (Underwood and Carr, 1972; Papadimitriou and Woods, 1975) and susceptible to a wide range of vasoactive compounds such as adrenaline and noradrenaline, acetylcholine, 5-hydroxytryptamine, bradykinin and kallikrein (Cater *et al.*, 1966; Cater and Taylor, 1966). It becomes, however, increasingly difficult to separate host and tumour vasculature and some of the alleged characteristics of tumour blood vessels may reflect non-specific local conditions within the tumour such as necrosis, haemorrhage and infection. Nevertheless, the details of blood flow within and near tumours is important since the vasculature represents a major channel of dissemination and, in consequence, an obvious target for measures to reduce metastatic spread. Folkman (1975) has discussed the development of possible "anti-angiogenesis" factors, and there is recent evidence that such factors may exist in normal cartilage (Brem and Folkman, 1975; Langer *et al.*, 1976)—a tissue which is strikingly resistant to invasion by extraneous tumour. It has been shown experimentally that the dioxopiperazin compound, ICRF 159, may prevent blood-borne metastases, possibly by acting on the vascular endothelium (Le Serve and Hellmann, 1972; Salsbury *et al.*, 1974; Atherton, 1975) though the underlying mechanisms are uncertain (cf. Peters, 1975). In particular, ICRF 159 has been shown to be effective in only certain tumour systems (cf. Pimm and Baldwin, 1975): it clearly does not act non-specifically on all tumour-associated capillary endothelium.

It is uncertain whether tumours have lymphatics within their substance (Futrell and Pories, 1975) though dilated lymph vessels are commonly seen in the adjacent stroma. The lymphatic and blood

vascular systems provide the major routes of tumour cell dissemination, and details of the process are given in the following sections.
It should, however, be noted that the separation between the two
systems is a convenient over-simplification. Some tumour cells,
initially distributed in lymphatics, will reach the blood vascular
system; and tumour cells, injected intravascularly, may cross the
interstitial space and enter the lymphatic compartment (Hilgard *et
al.*, 1972). Few groups of tumours in man metastasise exclusively by
one of these anatomic routes and, in some circumstances, haematogenous and lymphatic distribution seem to occur with near-equal
frequency.

The natural tendency of infiltrating tumour cells to invade local
vessels and body cavities may be enhanced by various assaults on the
primary tumour. Massage, incision, and partial removal of lesions
have long been known to facilitate tumour dissemination in
experimental animals (*see* Cameron, 1954). The possible hazard of
surgical biopsy of tumours in man has never been clarified but, in
general, there is little evidence that biopsy is harmful provided that
definitive treatment is not delayed.

III. Dissemination in Serous Cavities

The peritoneal, pleural and pericardial cavities may be invaded by
local tumour, either as a direct extension of the primary lesion or
from metastases which impinge on the cavity in question (Fig. 3).
The sequence of invasion, shedding of tumour cells into a body cavity
and their subsequent implantation has long been familiar (*see* Willis,
1973), but two points deserve further comment—the pattern of
distribution of metastatic tumour within body cavities, and the mode
of development of malignant effusions. Both have been investigated
chiefly in the peritoneum.

It is clear that the distribution of intraperitoneal metastases is not
random and that there are certain preferential sites for tumour
growth. These are the Pouch of Douglas in the pelvis, the root of the
mesentery, the superior aspect of the sigmoid mesocolon, the right
paracolic gutter and the omentum. A radiological investigation of a
series of patients with intraperitoneal malignancies by means of
peritoneography (Meyers, 1973) has extended these morphological
observations by showing that ascitic fluid exhibits definite flow
patterns determined by fluctuating intra-abdominal pressure and by
spontaneous intestinal movements. Most of the sites where intraperitoneal metastases are likely to occur coincide with sites of

"preferential, repeated or arrested flow of intraperitoneal fluid". Pleural metastases are most abundant on the diaphragmatic surface, in the costophrenic angles and along the paravertebral gutters; the basis for this distribution appears to be mechanical and there is no evidence of preferential sites of pleural involvement (Willis, 1973).

The mode of development of malignant ascites is ill-understood and the argument revolves round the relative importance of increased exudation of fluid and its decreased absorption from the peritoneal cavity. Excessive exudation of fluid may occur through the abnormally permeable vessels associated with local tumour; but the observations of Hirabayashi and Graham (1970) at laparotomy on patients with ascites from ovarian cancer indicate that there is considerable exudation of fluid from the *uninvolved* peritoneal surface. Indeed, these authors concluded that most of the ascitic fluid oozed from tumour-free peritoneal surfaces. The underlying mechanisms are unknown. Increased exudation may reflect the action of tumour-associated products which enhance vascular permeability, and such exudation would certainly be increased by any local inflammation. Ascitic fluid is rich in protein and its high osmotic pressure tends to militate against reabsorption from the peritoneal cavity. On the other hand, it is common experience that wide-spread intraperitoneal metastases may occur *without* ascites, and it has been proposed that the accumulation of ascites may (in part) reflect decreased peritoneal drainage due to obstruction of peritoneal lymphatics. Direct evidence for this view comes from studies on mediastinal lymphoscintigraphy in which a colloidal suspension of ^{99M}Tc-sulphur was injected intraperitoneally in patients with malignant ascites (Coates *et al.*, 1973). There was no evidence of any comparable lymphatic obstruction in control cases with non-malignant ascites. Clinical and experimental studies by Feldman (1975; also Feldman and Knapp, 1974) support the view that obstructed lymph flow is an important factor in the development of ascites. The role of intact sub-diaphragmatic lymphatic plexuses is stressed by Feldman, and experiments with a transplantable ovarian carcinoma in mice indicate that early and localized inflammatory changes in the diaphragm are quickly followed by increasing accumulation of ascitic fluid.

A recent experimental study by Fastaia and Dumont (1976), using Ehrlich-Lettré ascites tumour cells in mice, clearly implicates both the mechanisms postulated: first, and most importantly, a progressive increase in capillary permeability followed by increasing lymphatic obstruction.

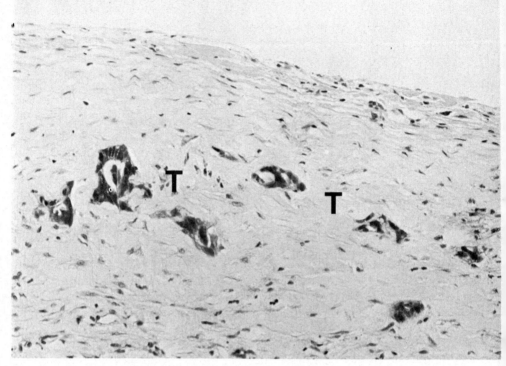

FIG. 3A. Metastatic growth in serous cavities. Female, 58. Small tumour deposits (T) from an ovarian adenocarcinoma which are seeding on the pelvic peritoneum. × 240

IV. Dissemination by Lymphatics

The lymphatic system provides the main mode of spread for carcinomas; it is also frequently involved by disseminating malignant melanoma, neuroblastoma and teratoma. Most sarcomas do not spread by lymphatics though lymph node deposits are sometimes encountered in rhabdomyosarcoma and leiomyosarcoma. Metastatic sarcomas in laboratory animals often spread to the draining lymph nodes.

The point of access is generally provided by small lymphatic vessels in the vicinity of the primary tumour. The larger lymphatic vessels which run close to venules and arterioles may also be involved. The "perineural lymphatics", described particularly near the prostate, bladder and pancreas, are thought to be perineural

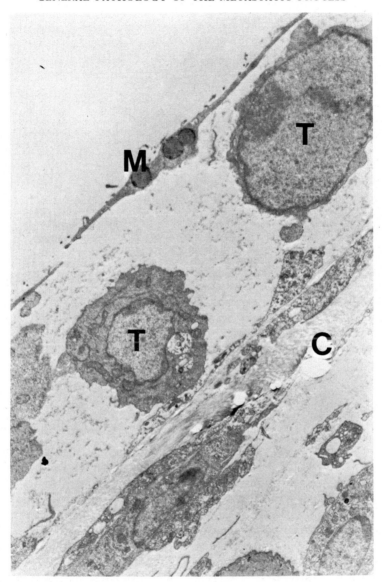

FIG. 3B. Metastatic growth in serous cavities. Experimental studies with a hamster lymphoma. Cells from a metastasising lymphoma implanted as an ascites in the peritoneal cavity. Tumour cells (T) have breached the mesothelial lining cells (M) and are infiltrating subperitoneal collagen fibres (C)

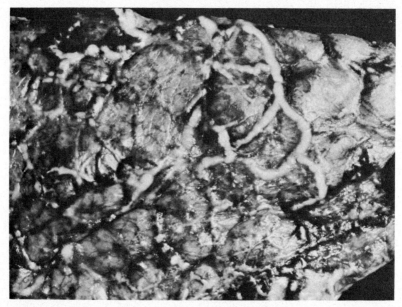

Fig. 4A. Neoplastic invasion of lymphatics. Female, 50. Carcinoma of breast. Subpleural lymphatics on the surface of the lung, infiltrated by metastatic tumour—"lymphangitis carcinomatosa". × 1.5

spaces rather than true lymphatic channels (Rodin *et al.*, 1967). Though broadly similar to capillaries in the blood vascular system, small lymphatics have certain characteristic features (Yoffey and Courtice, 1970). In some regions of the body they lack a basement membrane and show a high proportion of gap-junctions between adjacent endothelial cells. Both these features appear to be linked with the normal high permeability of lymphatic vessels; they may also be correlated with the apparent ease with which such vessels are invaded by tumour cells though the actual process of penetration has received little attention. The recent studies of Carr and his colleagues (Carr *et al.*, 1976) with the Rd/3 sarcoma in rats suggest that tumour cells enter through the gap-junctions and produce no visible damage to adjacent endothelium or collagen. Macrophages and lymphocytes migrate through the lymphatic wall in a similar manner. Inside the lymphatics, tumour cells enter the lymph stream—a low pressure flow system maintained jointly by extralymphatic forces provided by movements of skeletal muscles and pulsations transmitted by arteries, and by intrinsic rhythmic contractions of the vessels themselves (Hall, 1969). The neuropharmacology of normal lymph

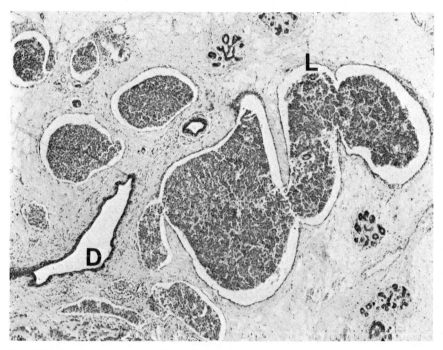

FIG. 4B. Neoplastic invasion of lymphatics. Female, 63. Carcinoma of breast. A local lymphatic vessel (L), sectioned at several points, contains clumps of invading carcinoma cells. D, normal breast duct. H & E × 55

flow is unknown and so, too, are the dynamic effects of an influx of relatively large particles such as tumour cells.

Tumour cells disseminate in lymphatics in two ways—in the form of emboli or as a solid continuous growth (Fig. 4). The latter process, known as *permeation*, was formerly regarded as the major mode of lymphatic spread. Based mainly on studies of advanced cancer of the breast, Sampson Handley proposed in 1906 a process of continuous growth of intralymphatic tumour outwards from the primary lesion. Subsequently this intralymphatic tumour was alleged to induce "the defensive process of perilymphatic fibrosis" (*sic*) which resulted in partial obliteration of the involved vessels. This view is now discarded, mainly because of the near-universal failure to demonstrate tumour cells in tissues intervening between a primary neoplasm and involved regional lymph nodes (Willis, 1973). An element of lymphatic permeation does, however, occur at certain sites, particularly in serous membranes such as the visceral pleura and mesentery, and in the thoracic duct; it may also be seen in the

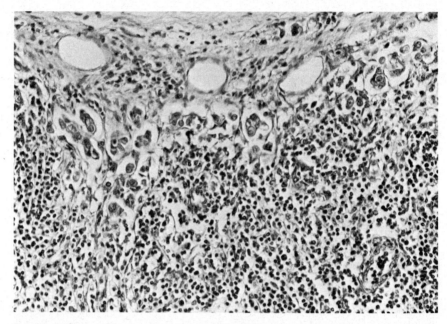

Fig. 5A. Tumour cells in lymph node sinuses. Female, 44. Carcinoma of breast. Tumour cells infiltrating the subcapsular sinus of an axillary lymph node. Note that the underlying pulp is intact. × 240

skin in association with slowly growing malignant melanomas (Willis, 1973).

Most tumour cells reach the regional lymph nodes in the afferent lymph as *emboli*, either in the form of single cells or as clumps. The time that may elapse since release of tumour cells from the primary lesion is likely to be variable, but little information is available on this point. Cells from a neuroblastoma, grafted as a solid implant into the anterior chamber of the eye in ABC mice, have been identified histologically in the draining lymph nodes 4 days after transplantation (Plenk *et al.*, 1954). Similar results have emerged from a more refined study by Wood and Carr (1974): 5×10^5 sarcoma cells (Rd/3), injected into the footpad of rats, regularly gave rise to a metastasis of about 0.5×10^5 cells in the draining popliteal lymph nodes after 4 days. Obviously, there is no comparable information for man.

Within lymph nodes, tumour cells are localized first in the subcapsular sinus, then in the interfollicular sinuses of the pulp and the medullary sinuses (Fig. 5). This predictable pattern is found in clinical material (Willis, 1973) and in more easily controlled

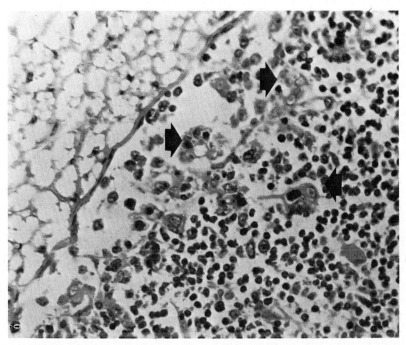

FIG. 5B. Tumour cells in lymph node sinuses. Experimental studies with a hamster lymphoma (NML). Axillary lymph nodes draining a 14-day old subcutaneous implant. Viable NML cells reach the regional node where they evoke an intense local response, one of the features of which is a large increase in sinus histiocytes (*see Chapter II*). Several macrophages are seen (arrows) which contain tumour cell debris

experimental conditions (Zeidman and Buss, 1954; Carter and Gershon, 1966, 1967; Ludwig and Titus, 1967). The anatomical arrangement of the sinus system in lymph nodes is well established (Yoffey and Courtice, 1970) and is consistent in man and animals. A vivid picture of the large subcapsular sinus is provided by the scanning electron microscope (Luk *et al.*, 1973) which shows a capacious channel broken up by an elaborate meshwork of long branching trabeculae, lined by lymphatic endothelium and macrophages.

A. *Non-immunological (Barrier) Function of Lymph Nodes*

The barrier function provided by lymph nodes against incoming tumour cells is open to question. First proposed by Virchow in 1860 (who observed that . . . "the lymph node elements lie crowded together like a charcoal filter"), this aspect of lymph node function appears to have lacked investigation for many years. Using rabbits, Zeidman and Buss (1954) injected cells from two squamous carcinomas—the V2 and the Brown-Pearce tumours—into afferent popliteal lymphatics, excised the popliteal nodes at intervals of 1 to 42 days later, and then killed the animals after 4 to 9 weeks. Their results suggested that tumour cells were efficiently trapped in the popliteal nodes for periods of about three weeks. The problem was re-analysed quantitatively in rabbits by Fisher and Fisher (1966, 1967a) who used a carefully monitored perfusion system and tumour cells labelled with isotopic chromium (^{51}Cr). Tumour cells, singly or in clumps, were regularly recovered from the cannulated efferent lymphatics. The authors concluded that "the majority of tumour cells entering a lymph node fail to maintain permanent residence". A number of important differences were established between the retention of tumour cells and of erythrocytes under the same experimental conditions. More erythrocytes were trapped than tumour cells (90% versus 40%); retention of red cells, but not of tumour cells, was dose-dependent; and retention of red cells, but not of tumour cells, was impaired by prior X-irradiation of the nodes and by local turpentine-induced intranodal inflammation.

The findings of the Fishers have not been universally accepted and various reservations may be put forward: the limited range of tumour cells and lymph nodes tested, the possible distortions in local lymph flow during cannulation and perfusion, and the fact that the lymph nodes had not been exposed to a local tumour growing in the drainage area as would have been the case in an intact animal. There is continuing debate about the extent and efficiency of the barrier function in different lymph nodes, in different animals, confronted by different tumours—see, for example, the experiments with mesenteric lymph nodes draining a transplanted caecal carcinoma in rats, described by Abe and Taneichi (1972). There are also discrepancies in the reported effects of local irradiation, though the detailed studies of Engesett (1966) support the view that trapping of tumour cells in lymph nodes is impaired by local irradiation. Lymphography, cortisone and exercise have been shown to compromise the barrier function of popliteal lymph nodes in rabbits (Engzell et al., 1968; Stoker, 1969). It is obvious that these manipulations, particularly local irradiation and cortisone treatment, are likely to act in many different ways and the effects on barrier function may be indirect.

Little is known of the barrier function of lymph nodes in man.

Fisch (1970) perfused lymph nodes in block dissections of the neck with red cells labelled with radioactive chromium. He advanced some evidence to suggest that pre-operative irradiation impaired the filtering activity of nodes in the treated area; but, given the artificial conditions under which these observations had to be made, their intepretation is difficult.

It is likely that the intrinsic properties of the tumour cells themselves may contribute to the efficacy (or otherwise) of trapping mechanisms in the regional lymph node. Nothing is known here, and experiments on the comparative *in vitro* adhesion of carcinoma and sarcoma cells to sinus elements (cf. Nicolson *et al.*, 1976) might be rewarding.

B. *Immunological Function of Lymph Nodes*

The immunological function of lymph nodes draining metastasising tumours, with particular reference to morphological changes, is discussed in *Chapter II* (*see also* Carter, 1975a, b).

C. *Fate of Retained Tumour Cells*

Once tumour cells are trapped in lymph nodes, various events may ensue.

(1) The cells may die, for metabolic reasons or possibly as a result of the activities of host inflammatory and immune cells (cf. Fig. 5B). Such responses are easier to study in experimental situations (Carter and Gershon, 1966, 1967; Ludwig and Titus, 1967) and it is not known whether tumour cells are killed by host elements in human lymph nodes; Willis (1973) doubts it

(2) The cells may survive in a dormant state without giving rise to a metastasis. If such a node is transplanted into a syngeneic recipient, local tumours will develop (Gershon *et al.*, 1967)—illustrating the important generalization that demonstration of living tumour cells in a node, or any other distant tissue, by means of bioassay is not necessarily synonymous with metastasis. It is unknown whether tumour cells can lie dormant in human lymph nodes.

(3) The cells may become established and grow. The acquisition of an adequate blood supply is essential and it is striking how rarely large nodal metastases from the common carcinomas in man show signs of ischaemia or infarction. The normal lymph node vasculature in animals is adaptable (Herman *et al.*, 1969, 1972) and it is probably

recruited to supply the developing focus of tumour. Angioneo-
genesis under the influence of tumour angiogenesis factor (TAF)
may also occur—*see* p. 7. It is not known whether, or for how long,
special features of lymph node vasculature such as the post-capillary
venules survive in nodes which are being replaced by metastatic
tumour—they have been described in nodes infiltrated by Hodgkin's
disease (Söderström and Norberg, 1974).

Growth of lymph node metastases is commonly progressive,
culminating in complete replacement of the normal pulp. Direct
extension through the capsule of the node may occur, a feature that
appears to be an important adverse prognostic discriminant in
axillary nodes involved by metastatic breast cancer (Fisher *et al.*,
1976). Capsular invasion is frequent in nodal metastases from
squamous carcinomas. On the other hand, it has sometimes been
suggested that established nodal metastases may partly regress. This
has been described in cervical nodes involved by thyroid carcinoma
and in axillary nodes containing mammary carcinoma (Crile, 1966;
Edwards *et al.*, 1972). Some of these alleged regressions may have
occurred in nodes which were enlarged because of reactive changes in
the absence of tumour deposits. More information is needed on this
important point.

D. *Late Consequences of Lymph Node Involvement*

As local lymph nodes are replaced by metastatic tumour, afferent
lymph flow will be increasingly deflected, carrying tumour cells to
fresh nodes (Fig. 6). Growing obstruction in the lymphatics and
intranodal sinuses will eventually lead to reversed lymph flow and
retrograde spread of tumour cells to distant and sometimes anomalous locations within the lymphoid system (*see* p. 36). Alterations in
lymphatic vasculature and lymph flow may also accrue from local
radiotherapy or surgery (Treidman and McNeer, 1963; Sherman
and O'Brian, 1967).

Tumour cells may disseminate into the blood vascular system* by
invading local vessels inside or outside the node or by traversing the
small lymphatico-venous communications that have been described

---

* There is experimental evidence that tumour cells may begin to pass from lymph nodes into
the blood stream at much earlier stages. In studies on barrier function which have already been
discussed, Fisher and Fisher (1967a) found that about half the tumour cells injected into the
afferent popliteal lymphatics were not trapped nor recovered in the efferent lymph. Though
unproven, it is probable that most of the tumour cells entered the blood. If this is the case and
the findings are of general validity in a clinical context, the implications are disturbing as
reassurance from "histologically uninvolved" lymph nodes may prove to be ill-founded.

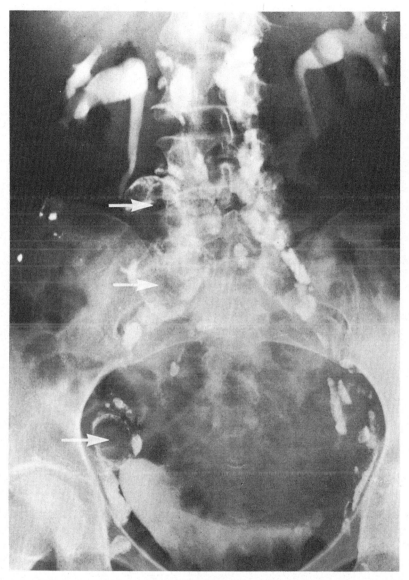

FIG. 6. Female, 61. Malignant melanoma on sole of right foot. Lymphangiogram taken 4 years after right mid-tarsal amputation and block dissection of right inguinal and external iliac nodes. Arrows point to enlarged nodes with big filling defects on right side, involving upper external iliac and para-aortic groups extending from the level of the second lumbar vertebra to the upper sacrum. (Illustration kindly supplied by Dr. J. S. Macdonald, Royal Marsden Hospital)

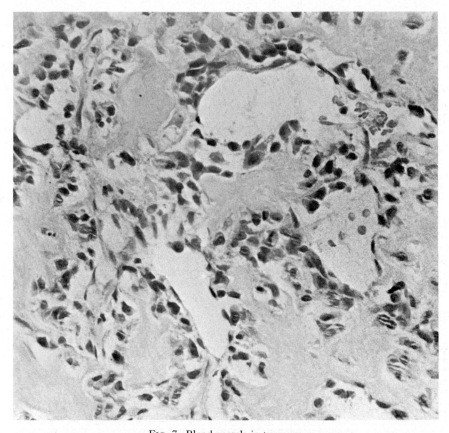

FIG. 7. Blood vessels in tumours
A. Male, 11. Osteogenic sarcoma of femur. Abnormal blood vessels which are partly lined by
tumour cells. × 240
B. (*facing page, top*) Same case. Normal vessel in thickened periosteum, near primary tumour,
invaded by neoplastic cells. × 240
C. (*facing page, lower*) Male, 34. Invasion of small radicle of testicular vein by teratoma. × 240

in animals and in man (Pressman *et al.*, 1962, 1964; Burn, 1968).
Once local lymphatic obstruction supervenes, these channels open
up and serve to link the lymphatic and blood vascular circuits.
Tumour cells may also enter the blood stream *via* large connecting
channels such as the thoracic duct.

V. Dissemination by the Blood Stream

Spread within the blood stream is particularly characteristic of
human sarcomas and choriocarcinoma. Neuroblastoma, malignant

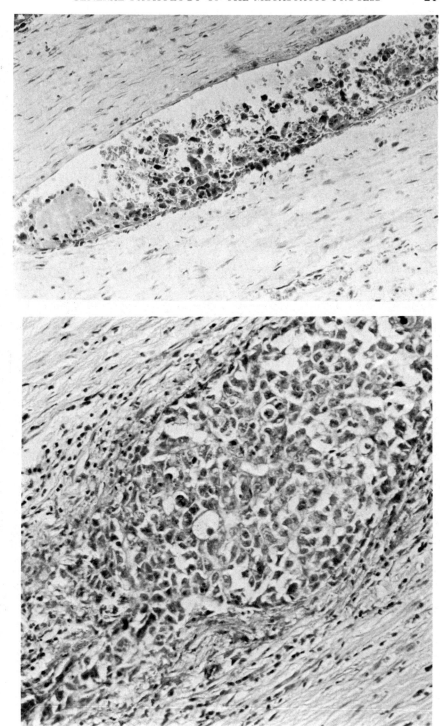

melanoma and teratomas tend to spread equally by haematogenous
and lymphatic routes and there is a variable element of blood-borne
spread in most disseminating carcinomas. Tumour cells may enter
the blood vascular system indirectly from lymphatic channels (v.s.)
or directly through vessels in or near the primary growth (Fig. 7).
Vessels within the substance of tumours are often abnormal (see p.
7); and in highly anaplastic lesions, particularly sarcomas, they may
consist of little more than irregular blood-filled spaces lined directly
by tumour cells (Willis, 1973). Perfusion through such structures is,
however, likely to be inadequate in many instances and it is probable
that the normally constituted venules and larger capillaries, lying in
the stroma near the growing edge of the primary tumour, provide the
main portal of entry. The mode of penetration by tumour cells into
such vessels is unknown. Arteries are rarely invaded, and some
elegant experiments in rabbits suggest that their apparent resistance
depends on intravascular pressure rather than the thickness of the
vessel wall. Shivas and Finlayson (1965) reported that Brown-Pearce
squamous carcinoma cells readily invaded and obliterated viable
segments of the femoral artery which were excluded from the
circulation by ligatures.

The time of vascular invasion is difficult to define. Romsdahl *et al.*
(1961) investigated the problem qualitatively using the Lewis lung
tumour implanted intramuscularly into C57B1 mice. The tumour-
bearing limbs were amputated in different groups on days 1 to 12 and
evidence of dissemination sought in venous blood (as free tumour
cells) and as macroscopic pulmonary metastases. Tumour cells were
identified in the blood as early as 24 hr after transplantation of the
graft. Although the viability of the circulating tumour cells was not
investigated and the effects of surgical trauma were not fully
controlled, the early appearance of tumour cells in the blood is
striking. More recently, this problem has been investigated quantitatively by Butler and Gullino (1975). These authors used a
mammary carcinoma (MTW 9) in Wistar-Furth rats which was
transplanted at the distal end of an ovarian pedicle and grown in a
subcutaneous pouch. The tumour was enclosed and effectively
isolated from surrounding tissues, and all the efferent blood from the
lesion drained into a single vein. It was found that, for tumours
weighing 2 to 4 gm, 3 to 4 million cells were shed into the blood per
day per gm of tissue. The cells released into the circulation were
rapidly cleared, giving rise to a 12-fold difference in the numbers of
cells in the venous blood draining the tumour and in the arterial side
of the circulation. Since about 10^6 cells are required to establish

100% of transplants with the MTW 9 tumour, it appears that enough cells are released *in vivo* in each 24 hr to transplant the lesion—though Butler and Gullino did not determine whether the cells were viable.

Tumour cells may be released into the blood stream as single cells or as small clumps, usually of around 7 or 8 cells. Recent experimental work suggests that single cells predominate but clumps appear to be particularly important in favouring subsequent metastatic growth. B16 melanoma cells injected intravenously in small clumps into C57B1 mice have a greater tendency to form deposits than the same number of single melanoma cells (Fidler, 1973b). Tumour cell clumps are a consistent finding in venous blood draining implants of the metastasising T241 fibrosarcoma in C57B1 mice and, once again, injection of T241 cells in clumps of 6 or 7 produced a greater number of deposits than the same number of single cells (Liotta *et al.*, 1974, 1976).

A. *Circulating Tumour Cells*

Tumour cells in the circulation, probably first described by Ashworth in 1869, have been extensively studied in man (Griffiths and Salsbury, 1965; Malmgren, 1968; Salsbury, 1975). They may occur as single cells or as small clumps (Fig. 8); they tend to be more commonly found in patients with sarcomas than carcinomas; and they are more readily demonstrated during the later stages of the disease. The proportion of positive results depends on many variables such as the site of sampling (venous effluent from the primary tumour itself or a peripheral vein), the time and frequency of sampling (especially in relation to any surgical or other manipulative procedure), the amount of blood taken, and the method used to concentrate the cells. Once identified—and accurate identification can be exceedingly difficult—it has to be conceded that the practical significance of demonstrating circulating tumours cells is small. There is near-unanimous agreement that such a demonstration is of little prognostic significance, irrespective of the site or type of primary tumour (Candar *et al.*, 1962; Griffiths and Salsbury, 1965; Griffiths *et al.*, 1973). It is possible that the circulating cells are post-mitotic or have a limited life span, or that for some reason they are unable to adhere to vascular endothelium. Attempts to establish such cells in culture *in vitro* have been unsuccessful.

An unavoidable limitation of studies on circulating tumour cells in man is that they are entirely qualitative. Several quantitative

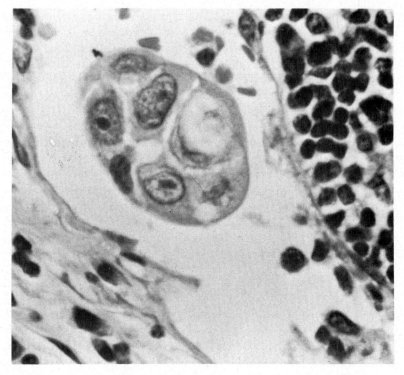

FIG. 8. Intravascular tumour cells
A. Male, 57. Carcinoma of bronchus. Tumour cell embolus in small vessel. × 1000
(Illustration kindly supplied by Dr. A. J. Salsbury)

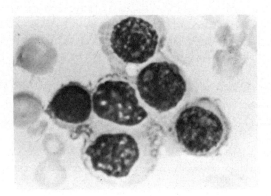

B. Female, 54. Carcinoma of breast. Tumour cells isolated from venous blood concentrate.
× 1000 (Illustration kindly supplied by Dr. A. J. Salsbury)

investigations have been made in laboratory animals by the simple expedient of injecting known numbers of tumour cells directly into the circulation (e.g. Baserga *et al.*, 1960; Fisher and Fisher, 1967b; Fidler, 1970, 1973b). It is commonly found that there is a high death rate among injected tumour cells with a surviving, proliferating fraction of <1% though there is a broadly consistent dose-response relationship between the numbers of tumour cells injected and the eventual number of deposits of "secondary" growth. Work by Fidler (1973b) has suggested an unexpected supportive role for dead and dying tumour cells in a system involving intravenous injection of B16 melanoma cell lines into syngeneic C57B1 mice. The inclusion in some inocula of known numbers of melanoma cells killed by γ-irradiation was associated with a consistently enhanced yield of tumour deposits in the lungs. Similar results were obtained when the irradiated tumour cells were replaced by dead C57B1 embryonic cells.

Several animal systems have been described where there is a progressively growing primary tumour (autochthonous or transplanted) and many circulating cells, but no metastases (Kim, 1966; Gershon *et al*, 1967; Wexler *et al.*, 1969; Crile *et al.*, 1971). The circulating cells are clearly viable as transfer of whole blood gives rise to local tumours in the recipients. The failure of these cells to generate metastases may be due to immune and other host responses, a topic that is discussed in Section VII and also in *Chapters II* and *VI*.

B. *Arrested Tumour Cells*

Morphologists at the beginning of the century described tumour cell emboli attached to capillary walls within a thrombus (*see* Willis, 1973). More recently, the dynamics of tumour cell arrest were investigated in a classic study by Wood (1958). V2 squamous carcinoma cells were injected intra-arterially in rabbit ears and subsequent events, visualized in ear chambers, were recorded by continuous cine-micrography. Small clumps of tumour cells, generally 6 to 10, stuck to vascular endothelium where they were enmeshed in a clot of fibrin and platelets. Local endothelial defects then developed in the vicinity of polymorphs which were caught up in the thrombus. The leucocytes passed through into the interstitial space. Within 3 to 6 hours, the tumour cells had followed. The sequence of events is summarized in Fig. 9. Wood concluded that the initial site of adhesion was not determined by vessel diameter, the rate of blood flow or by vasomotor activity but he suggested that the

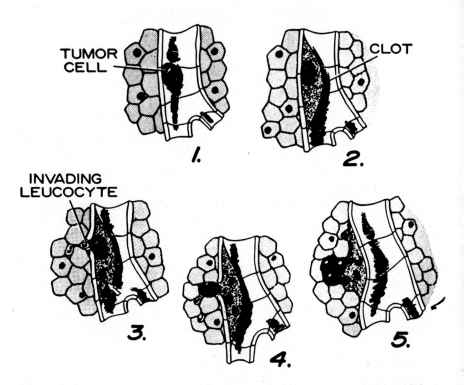

FIG. 9. The traditional sequence of events whereby intravascular tumour cells establish an extravascular focus: 1. Clump of tumour cells adheres to vessel wall; 2. A clot forms; 3. Leucocytes, enmeshed in the clot, breach the vessel wall; 4. Tumour cells follow; 5. Tumour cells accumulate in the adjacent extravascular space. This scheme of events summarizes the original description made by Sumner Wood (1958) with V2 tumour cells in the rabbit ear chamber. Several details of Wood's scheme are now disputed—see text. (Illustration reproduced from Fisher, B. and Fisher, E. R. (1962), *Surg. Clin. N. Amer.*, **42**, 335, by permission of the authors and publishers)

process was favoured by the innate stickiness of tumour cell surfaces and their capacity to liberate thromboplastin-like substances. The importance of local intravascular thrombosis is suggested by several experimental studies in which the incidence of metastases was generally diminished by treatment with anticoagulant, fibrinolytic or thrombocytopenic agents (for references *see* Brown, 1973).

Some of the observations summarized above are now disputed and the underlying mechanisms of tumour cell arrest are still obscure.

(1) Interaction between tumour cell and endothelium involves the interplay of highly complex physical forces in which electrostatic and viscous barriers, inimical to contact, are pitted against kinetic factors

such as the radial velocity of the circulating tumour cell. These and several other parameters are still to be clarified in simplified *in vitro* models, and their operation in an *in vivo* situation remains largely theoretical (Weiss, 1967, 1973, 1976). It is, however, now possible to quantitate *in vivo* the adhesiveness of circulating leucocytes to the walls of vessels in the hamster cheek pouch and mouse mesentery (Atherton and Born, 1972, 1973), and this technique could be adapted to the study of intravascular tumour cells.

(2) It is uncertain how far the arrested tumour cells themselves activate thrombus formation. Holyoke *et al.* (1972) assayed thromboplastin activity released into the medium from short-term cultures of the murine Lewis T241 sarcoma. They found more thromboplastin/mg of total cell protein in fluids from *control* cultures of embryonic epithelium and embryonic fibroblasts. The authors concluded that although thromboplastin activity is associated with tumour cells it is not a specific characteristic of them. Hilgard (1973) suggests that adherent tumour cells inflict "minimal endothelial damage", resulting in leakage into the plasma of cytoplasmic contents which activate the clotting mechanism.

(3) The central importance of the fibrin clot is disputed. Aggregates of tumour cells may sometimes be seen attached to vessels lacking platelets and/or fibrin (Ludatscher *et al.*, 1967; Jones *et al.*, 1971; Cotmore and Carter, 1973), though it has been suggested that fibrin may be present in only very small amounts and that the platelet-fibrin complex disintegrates after a few hours (Chew *et al.*, 1976). There is some evidence that the amount of fibrin present may reflect in a purely non-specific fashion the extent of local endothelial damage; total loss of endothelium will result in loss of fibrinolytic activity (Warren and Vales, 1972).

(4) The antimetastatic effects of some anticoagulants, claimed by several workers, is also being questioned. A detailed study of the effects of warfarin on spontaneous lung metastases from the KHT sarcoma, implanted intramuscularly in C3H mice, provides convincing evidence that this anticoagulant reduces the numbers of lung deposits and acts solely on the host's clotting mechanism (Brown, 1973); but more problematic are the results from experiments with the defibrinating agent "Arvin" and (especially) with heparin. Single doses of Arvin, a material derived from Malayan pit-viper venom, increased the number of deposits from the B16 melanoma and the MCGI-SS sarcoma, injected intravenously (Hagmar, 1972a). Analogous increases in deposits from these two tumours have been described in animals anticoagulated with heparin (Hagmar, 1970,

1972b; Hagmar and Norrby, 1970). The results with heparin emphasize that the effects of anticoagulants are complex and, in several experimental protocols, may impinge equally on host clotting mechanisms and on the tumour cells themselves. The effects which heparin may exert on tumour cells include alterations in membrane function, cell volume, adhesiveness, electrophoretic mobility and formation of cell aggregates and cell-to-cell contacts of various kinds (Hagmar and Norrby, 1970; Hagmar, 1972b; Brown, 1973). Given this complex and diverse mode of action, it is essential that experiments on the effects of anticoagulants on metastasis should include groups in which the tumour cells and the recipient animals are each exposed separately to the anticoagulant being tested.

Particular attention has been focussed on the platelet component in tumour cell-associated thrombi. Hilgard (1973) has demonstrated that intravascular injection of Walker carcinosarcoma cells in rats is quickly followed by thrombocytopenia, due to a loss of circulating platelets as a result of thrombus formation around tumour cell emboli in the lungs. The degree of thrombocytopenia was linearly related to the numbers of tumour cells injected. The same platelet changes were elicited when dead Walker tumour cells or isolated tumour cell membranes were injected. Hilgard found no evidence of platelet aggregation by Walker tumour cells though this observation conflicts with previous findings of Warren (1970). Measures that establish thrombocytopenia before tumour cells are introduced into the body exert an antimetastatic effect which can be reversed by a platelet infusion (Gasic et al., 1968).

It is important to clarify the effects of anticoagulants on the metastatic process in view of the potential therapeutic implications. There is some experimental (Ryan et al.,1968) and clinical (Michaels, 1964; Elias et al., 1973) evidence which suggests that long-term anticoagulation, most commonly with dicoumarin drugs, may decrease the incidence of metastatic disease; but more information is needed with specified regimes and specified tumours, given at carefully defined phases of the disease, before any firm conclusion can be drawn. Combinations of anticoagulant and cytotoxic therapy should also be appraised.

Variations in the endothelium have received little attention. Topics which merit consideration include regional variation in the fine structure of endothelium, its adhesiveness and other surface properties, its susceptibility to sustain (and repair) damage, and its fibrinolytic activity.

C. *Fate of Arrested Tumour Cells*

Once tumour cells are attached to the vessel wall, various consequences may arise.

(1) Some cells, stuck loosely to the endothelium, may either become detached and shed into the circulation or die (Wood, 1971).

(2) Having acquired (in many cases) a protective capsule of fibrin and/or platelets, the tumour cell embolus is covered by regenerating endothelium and may then undergo varying degrees of organization. Seemingly inactive tumour cell emboli, enclosed in many endothelial layers, have been described in the walls of pulmonary vessels (Ludatscher *et al.*, 1967).

(3) Tumour cells, with or without an endothelial covering, begin to infiltrate the vessel wall. Two different mechanisms have been described.

(i) The most commonly held view is that tumour cells send out pseudopodia which penetrate between endothelial cells in a manner akin to extravasating leucocytes (Fig. 10). The time taken to breach the lining basement membrane and enter the extravascular compartment is variable. Jones *et al.* (1971) cite a figure of 24 to 48 hr for Walker carcinosarcoma cells, injected intravenously, to escape from the pulmonary vasculature in rats—considerably longer than the 5 to 8 hr taken by V2 squamous carcinoma cells to traverse vessels in the rabbit ear chamber (Wood, 1958). It is feasible that different tumour cells may penetrate different vessels at different speeds, but there are certain other discrepancies between Wood's original observations and the more recent electron microscopy studies. The endothelial defects, described by Wood at low-power magnification, have not been recorded in other experimental systems and the importance of previous leucocyte emigration has not been confirmed. It is postulated that tumour cells themselves inflict minute local lesions sufficient to allow their egress, but it must be conceded that their mode of production is quite unknown. Tumour cells may release proteinases or hyaluronidase; alternatively, they may elaborate vasoactive substances which induce contraction of endothelial cells and consequent widening of intercellular junctions.

(ii) A different mechanism has been proposed by Chew and his colleagues (Chew *et al.*, 1976) in a detailed ultrastructural

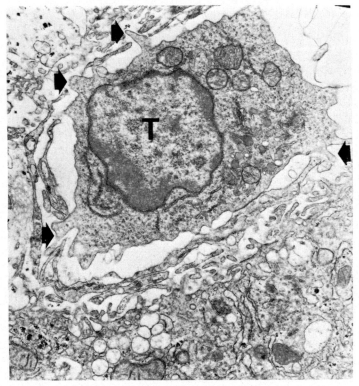

Fig. 10. Experimental studies with a metastasising hamster lymphoma. A tumour cell (T) lies
in an hepatic sinusoid. Note the pseudopodia (arrows) which extend between the endothelial
lining cells. There is no fibrin clot and no associated accumulation of leucocytes (cf. Fig. 9)

investigation using Walker carcinosarcoma cells in rats. This
work is outstanding for the fact that the escape of intravascular
tumour cells was studied at four different sites—lungs, liver,
brain and pituitary gland; a broadly similar pattern of events
was found at each. The authors were unable to demonstrate
diapedesis of tumour cells, akin to emigrating leucocytes, and
they described a process of attrition by tumour cells, "first of
endothelium and then of basement membrane at multiple
points". They summarize the process neatly by saying that . . .
"The tumour cell does not vacate the vessel, it destroys it".

It is obvious that these two mechanisms of tumour cell egress are
widely divergent, and further work is required to clarify the issue.

VI. Establishment and Growth of Extravascular Tumour in Distant Sites

This important phase in the metastatic process is particularly ill-understood, but it is possible to reconstruct a tentative series of events.

Free tumour cells, lacking an organized stroma, are likely to be vulnerable. Many will die, either from metabolic causes or possibly as a result of local inflammatory and immune defences. Some extravasated tumour cells may cross the interstitial space and enter lymphatics (Fisher and Fisher, 1968; Wood, 1971; Hilgard *et al.*, 1972). Once survivors from this initial phase acquire a stroma, their future development is more secure.

Existing vasculature may be recruited and perhaps augmented by local inflammation (*see* p. 45), and the tumour cells may stimulate new vascular proliferation by release of angiogenesis factors (v.s.). Distinction between these two processes is difficult in man but evidence of tumour-directed angiogenesis may perhaps be adduced from the interesting ultrastructural observations of Hirano and Zimmerman (1972) who described a renal carcinoma, metastasising to the brain, whose blood vessels showed a fenestrated arrangement characteristic of renal rather than cerebral vasculature. More information along these lines is needed. The experimental observations of Folkman and his colleagues (*see* Gimbrone *et al.*, 1972, 1973) are important in this context. These workers have shown that if tumour cells are in a location which is inadequately vascularized, the chances of their progressive growth are small. Fragments of the Brown-Pearce squamous carcinoma, implanted into the normally avascular anterior chamber of the eye of rabbits, acquire few blood vessels and grow to only a limited extent even though the constituent tumour cells remain fully viable and can be labelled with ^{3}H-thymidine. If such tumour nodules are then re-transplanted a short distance into the vascular milieu of the iris, rapid growth ensues. A similar picture is seen with the V2 squamous carcinoma or a mouse ependymoblastoma, transplanted into the vitreous of the rabbit or the dog (Brem *et al.*, 1976). The tumours form small unvascularized cell aggregates until they impinge on the retinal surface: "explosive growth into a large vascularized mass" then ensues.

Products released by tumour cells which aid the establishment of a new focus of growth have been particularly studied in relation to skeletal metastases (Fig. 11). The products include parathyroid hormone, possibly vitamin D and some of its metabolites, pros-

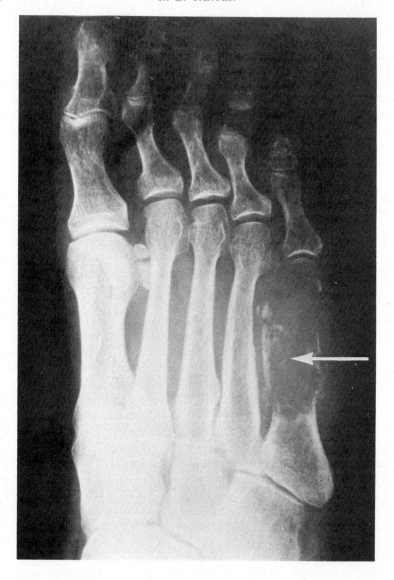

Fig. 11. Skeletal metastases
A. Male, 65. Oat cell carcinoma of bronchus. Osteolytic deposit in fifth metatarsal (arrow), almost completely destroying the shaft and head
B. (*facing page, top*) Male, 71. Carcinoma of prostate. Widespread osteoblastic deposits in pelvis and spine.
(Both radiographs kindly supplied by Dr. J. S. Macdonald, Royal Marsden Hospital)
C. (*facing page, lower*) Female, 67. Adenocarcinoma of bronchus. Decalcified lumbar vertebra in which normal bone marrow elements (B) are partly replaced by a large metastatic deposit (T)

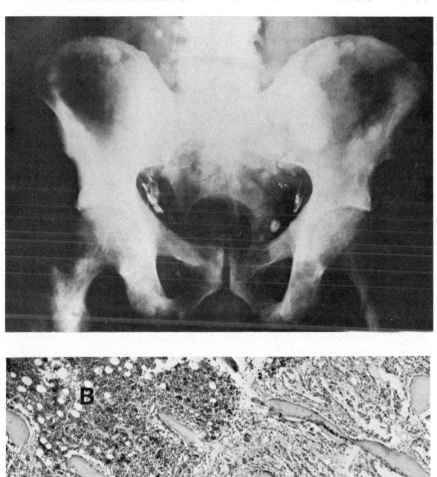

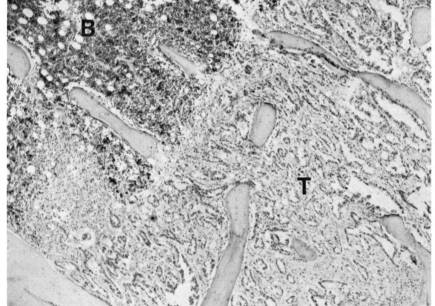

taglandins and osteoclastic activating factor (OAF). The Walker carcinosarcoma in rats, a mouse fibrosarcoma and also certain human breast cancers release prostaglandins which can be demonstrated by *in vitro* bioassay systems such as the local resorption of mouse calvarial bones (Powles *et al.*, 1973; Tashjian *et al.*, 1974). OAF has been described in supernatant fluids from cultures of cells from Burkitt lymphoma and from multiple myeloma but not from other lymphoid or haematopoietic neoplasms (Mundy *et al.*, 1974a, b). Elaboration of these humoral agents is far from being a specific characteristic of neoplastic cells. Prostaglandin-like material is released in the vicinity of non-neoplastic and inflammatory lesions such as dental cysts (Harris *et al.*, 1973), and the question of a multiple origin of prostaglandins—from tumour cells and from host inflammatory cells—obviously arises. OAF has been described in association with normal lymphocytes transformed by phytohaemag-glutinin (PHA). As far as prostaglandins are concerned, the immediate problems seem to be to identify the range of pros-taglandins produced, to identify their cell(s) of origin and to clarify their mode of action—particularly as there is now evidence that prostaglandin synthesis may be a necessary intermediary step in another osteolytic process, mediated by the enzyme collagenase (*see* Dowsett *et al.*, 1976). At a clinical level, more detailed comparative studies of prostaglandin synthesis are required of tumours which do, or do not, give rise to osteolytic metastases (Bennett *et al.*, 1975; Powles *et al.*, 1976). The genesis of osteoblastic, as opposed to osteolytic, metastases remains unclear, particularly as osteolytic and osteoblastic deposits may co-exist in the same patient and even within the same bone (Willis, 1973).

Little is known of the cell kinetics of early metastases. Since the growth fraction tends to decline as the tumour cell population increases in size, micrometastases should theoretically be parti-cularly sensitive to cell cycle-specific drugs (Schabell, 1975). This means that the drug-response of cells in primary and secondary tumours may differ. In man, it is rarely feasible to compare cell kinetics of primary and secondary neoplasms in the same patient. Charbit *et al.* (1971) compromised by comparing the mean doubling times of primary cancers of the breast and bronchus with secondaries of the same histological type in different patients. They found that the doubling times in the metastases were shorter by a factor of about 1·5 to 2. This observation might be regarded as consonant with the emergence of a clone of cells within the tumour with an enhanced malignant potential (cf. Fidler, 1973a); opposed to such a view is the general finding that karyotypes in metastatic tumours are either the same as, or are exactly double, the chromosome complement of the primary lesion. It is possible that metastases from a single primary may grow at different rates in different sites, but too few cases have been investigated to put such an observation on a firm footing. Equally, metastases derived from the same tumour but growing at different sites may vary in their susceptibility to chemotherapy (Conzelman and Springer, 1969; *see* also Slack and Bross, 1975): an example is provided by the divergent responses of skeletal and soft tissue deposits to chemotherapy that are sometimes seen in disseminated cancers of the breast.

Histologically, most established metastases resemble their tumour of origin. Secondary neoplasms that appear morphologically more differentiated are infrequent, but examples in man include metastases from squamous carcinomas of the nasopharynx and also teratomas. The latter may occasionally show signs of morphological maturation. Secondary tumours which are less well-differentiated than the corresponding primary are somewhat more common. Large discrepancies in either direction in the appearance of primary and secondary growths may cause much diagnostic confusion, sometimes raising the question of multiple primary tumours. Some metastases retain evidence of functional as well as morphological differentiation, judged by continuing synthesis of mucins or more complex, biologically active products such as hormones or carcinofoetal antigens.

Once clinically apparent, metastases tend to grow progressively; but there are rare circumstances where growth may be arrested or regression (complete or partial) supervenes. So-called *spontaneous regressions* are best documented for renal carcinoma, malignant melanoma, neuroblastoma and choriocarcinoma (Everson and Cole, 1966). The underlying mechanisms are unknown but the obvious points of enquiry are a change in tumour cell kinetics, vascular factors and immunological responses.

A different variant of metastatic growth is illustrated by the phenomenon of *dormancy* where metastases from certain tumours— notably breast, kidney and uveal tract—may manifest themselves many years after seemingly successful treatment of the primary lesion. Dormancy has been reproduced experimentally by Fisher and Fisher (1959) who injected small numbers of Walker carcinosarcoma cells (50–250) into the hepatic portal vein of rats. Few or no local deposits developed for periods of up to 20 weeks, but numerous tumours appeared after laparotomy and handling the liver (sham hepatectomy) and also after treatment with the hepatotoxic agent chloroform. These results have been broadly confirmed by Sugarbaker *et al.* (1971), using larger numbers of Walker tumour cells in the same allogeneic system; but it is interesting that attempts to repeat the observations with a syngeneic benzpyrene-induced sarcoma in Fisher rats were unsuccessful. The basis of dormancy is unknown. The kinetics of the tumour cells themselves may, for obscure reasons, have undergone some radical change such as a massive switch into a prolonged (non-proliferative) G_0 phase. The elegant studies of Folkman and his colleagues, discussed earlier, indicate the important contribution made by *local vasculature* in determining the development, extent and duration of the dormant site. *Trauma*, which is known to stimulate dormant tumour cells, may act in part by increasing regional blood flow and proliferation of new vessels. Immunological factors may also be incriminated (cf. Gershon *et al*, 1968; *see also Chapter VI*). Finally, it should be noted that non-neoplastic cells may lie dormant. Taptiklis (1968) showed that normal dissociated thyroid cells, injected intravenously into NZO/B1 mice, persist in the lungs for up to one year but remain capable of responding to thyrotrophic hormone by proliferating and forming follicles. In a later study, Taptiklis (1969) showed that thyroid cells obtained from goitrogen-induced tumours, from hyperplastic glands and from normal glands shared a common capacity to penetrate the pulmonary vascular endothelium in mice and establish deposits in the perivascular lung parenchyma.

VII. Localization of Metastatic Tumour

A. *Lymphatic Metastases*

The distribution of most metastases deriving from lymph-borne tumour cells is broadly explicable on mechanical and anatomical grounds—though it should not be concluded that our current knowledge of the detailed anatomy of lymph drainage from certain sites is complete. (As one example, pathologists frequently encounter metastatic carcinoma in pancreatic lymph nodes at autopsy in patients dying with cancers of the breast or bronchus: the relevant routes of lymphatic drainage are not clear). Involvement of the proximal set of regional lymph nodes is usual, followed in many cases by spread to contiguous lymph nodes in the next anatomical group (cf. Fig. 6). Orderly lymphatic spread may equally involve non-nodal structures such as parenchymal organs—liver and lungs—which lie within the lymphatic drainage area. Anomalies arise when deposits of tumour distort the local pattern of lymph flow or reverse it. Retrograde lymphatic spread may, for example, be responsible for involvement of distant or contralateral nodes. Modifications of lymphatic dissemination may follow obstruction of the cysterna chyli or thoracic duct; one well known consequence is the appearance of metastases in the supraclavicular nodes from primary intra-abdominal carcinomas.

B. *Haematogenous Metastases*

The pattern of metastases generated by blood-borne tumour cells presents more difficult problems, mainly because of the inconstant relation between the site where tumour cells are first trapped in the circulation and the sites where metastases ultimately develop. The association between initial trapping of intravascular tumour cells and eventual metastatic tumour is clear in the liver, which receives the venous drainage from the hepatic portal system, and in the lungs which drain the caval system. Both sites form effective catchment areas, and both are often involved by haematogenous metastases. The mode of involvement of other tissues—the axial skeleton, kidneys, adrenals, skin, brain—by blood-borne tumour emboli is more problematic. The importance of retrograde venous spread is disputed, particularly from unobstructed veins where Willis (1973) finds the evidence for such a process "unconvincing". Also disputed is the role of the paravertebral venous plexuses of Batson which have been implicated as an important route for intravascular tumour cells—particularly from cancers of the prostate, breast and perhaps thyroid—to gain access to the axial skeleton. Willis tends to regard this route as a minor one but others consider it to be an important channel for metastatic involvement (Drury *et al.*, 1964). Paravertebral venous spread has been reproduced experimentally with Walker and V2 tumour cells injected into the femoral veins of rats and rabbits (Coman and de Long, 1951). Van den Brenk *et al.* (1975) have shown that a proportion of Walker tumour cells, injected into the tail veins of rats, is regularly trapped in the ramifications of the venous system of the tail, hindquarters and pelvis where they give rise to solid tumours in the general distribution of the paravertebral venous plexuses.

1. *Access to the systemic circulation*

Various factors may be involved in situations where the site of development of metastatic deposits cannot satisfactorily be explained on the basis of initial intravascular trapping.

(1) The early morphologists recognized that tumour cells some-times traversed the pulmonary capillaries in experimental animals and entered the systemic circulation. This process was described by Takahashi in 1915 who made the important additional observation that transpulmonary spread occurred only with certain types of tumour. Zeidman and Buss (1952) injected various tumour cells—the V2 and Brown–Pearce squamous carcinomas and the Walker carcinosarcoma—into the ear veins of rabbits and simultaneously collected aortic blood and injected it intravenously into fresh recipients. Tumours developed in these recipients in 3 to 5 weeks with the Brown-Pearce tumour cells giving the highest incidence of "metastatic" lesions—an interesting reflection of its aggressive behaviour *in vivo*. Later cine-micrographic studies of V2 and Brown-Pearce tumour cells injected into the mesenteric arteries of rabbits graphically showed the tumour cells distorting and squeezing through the capillaries to enter the venous circulation (Zeidman, 1961). Trans-capillary movement was most marked in the (more malignant) Brown-Pearce cells even though they were generally larger than V2 cells. More recent cine-micrographs of various injected tumour cells traversing capillaries in the mesentery of the rat have been published by Sato and Suzuki (1972).

(2) Studies with radioactive labelled tumour cells* indicate that cells, initially trapped in the pulmonary circulation, are often redistributed (Fidler, 1970, 1973b; Brown, 1973; Weston *et al.*, 1974). This redistribution may occur early, within the first ten minutes after injection; it is not seen with dead tumour cells. The mechanisms are not clear but the sequence proposed by Fidler (1973b) is interesting, albeit unproven. Mechanical obstruction by impacted emboli induces vasoconstriction which spreads. A phase of pulmonary hypertension supervenes. Anastamotic channels open in response to anoxia, and some tumour cells are shunted towards the systemic circulation.

(3) Established pulmonary metastases may shed cells into the systemic circulation. Willis (1973) emphasizes that such metases may be minute and missed at a cursory examination.

* The use of radioactive-labelled tumour cells has often been mentioned in this chapter. It is important to note some of the technical limitations of such work, particularly the problems posed by the use of isotopes such as ^{51}Cr and ^{3}H which can be re-utilized after the death of the cell. "Contamination" by labelled stromal cells should also be borne in mind. Current opinion favours the use of ^{125}I-IUDR as a marker. A critical appraisal of the technical problems is given by Fidler (1970, 1976).

2. Tumour cells in the systemic circulation

Tumour cells reaching the systemic circulation are presumably distributed in a generalized fashion; yet one of the cardinal features of metastatic growth in man and in animals is the non-random nature of organ involvement. Metastases do not develop at all sites indiscriminately; different tumours often give rise to different and sometimes distinctive patterns of organ involvement; and some sites apparently escape. The proposition that certain structures are inherently "resistant" to metastatic involvement is perhaps over-emphasized, particularly as methods of demonstrating metastatic tumour are crude. The careful study of Berge (1974) illustrates, for example, that splenic metastases are not rare: an incidence of 7% was found in an unselected autopsy series of 312 cancer cases. Berge quotes a remark from Shaw Dunn that "the anticipated negative result is usually confirmed when examination of the organ is restricted to a single slice and a sceptical glance". In experimental animals, various tumours implanted directly into "resistant" tissues such as spleen or skeletal muscle grow as well as in susceptible sites such as the liver (de Long and Coman, 1950). Given generalized distribution of tumour cells in the systemic circulation, it appears that a major factor is the degree of access to peripheral tissues: in "resistant" sites, tumour cells are either not arrested or are unable to escape out into the extravascular compartment (Coman, 1953). These (implied) regional variations in vascular structure and function have been discussed previously.

Mechanistic considerations of this kind provide only a partial explanation of the localization of metastatic tumour, and several other factors must be considered. They include the local tissue environment, extraneous factors such as trauma and irradiation, inflammatory and immunological responses, and intrinsic attributes of the tumour cells themselves.

3. The local tissue environment

The view that certain tissues might provide particularly fertile "soil" for potential metastatic growth was proposed by Paget in 1889. It is, as Cameron remarked in 1954, a hypothesis that "has led to little action though much speculation". The literature is large and variable in quality but there are several studies which merit consideration. Some examples will be briefly cited.

(1) Lucké *et al.* (1952) injected equal numbers of V2 squamous carcinoma cells in the femoral vein or hepatic portal vein of rabbits.

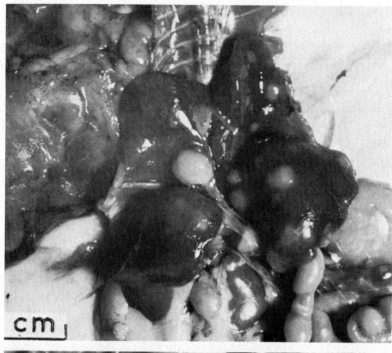

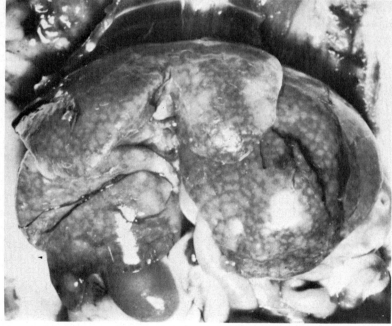

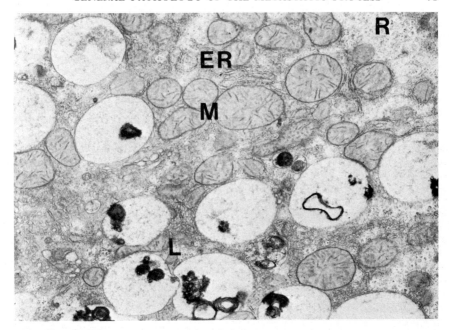

Consistently more deposits of tumour developed in the liver than the lungs.

(2) Kinsey (1960) found that subcutaneous grafts of the S91 melanoma in DBA2 mice metastasised exclusively to the lungs. This selectivity persisted when lung tissue was transplanted into the muscles of the thigh. Grafts of several other DBA2 tissues—liver, kidney, spleen, thyroid, heart, skin—were never involved by metastatic tumour.

(3) Extensive studies by the Fishers on the growth of Walker tumour cells injected intraportally in rats (Fisher and Fisher, 1968)

Fig. 12. "Soil" factors and metastasis. Hepatic metastases in hamsters treated with the non-ionic detergent Triton WR-1339
A. (*facing page*) Liver metastases, derived from a solid subcutaneous implant of a metastasising lymphoma, in: a normal hamster (*above*) and a hamster treated with Triton WR (*below*). Both animals killed 18 days after transplantation of the tumour. B. (*above*) Effects of Triton WR on hepatocyte lysosomes; normal hamster; 18 days. Several lysosomes (L) are shown: they appear enlarged and vacuolated and contain electron-dense material, sometimes arranged in whorls. Electron microscope autoradiographs have shown that Triton WR is selectively accumulated in the lysosomes. Other intracellular structures such as mitochondria (M), endoplasmic reticulum (ER) and ribosomes (R) appear normal. × 16,000

Overleaf
C. (*see page 42*) Tumour-bearing hamster treated with Triton WR; 18 days. Several tumour cells (T) infiltrating hepatic parenchymal cells which show marked lysosomal vacuolation. × 16,000
D. (*see page 42*) Tumour-bearing hamster; no Triton WR; 18 days. A single tumour cell surrounded by apparently normal hepatocytes. × 16,000

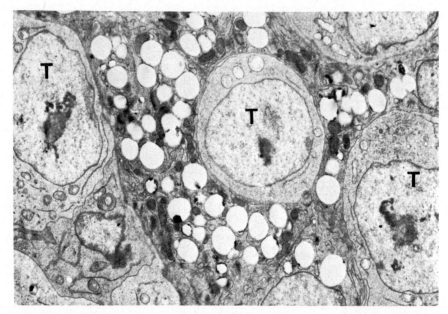

FIG. 12C. For legend *see* page 41

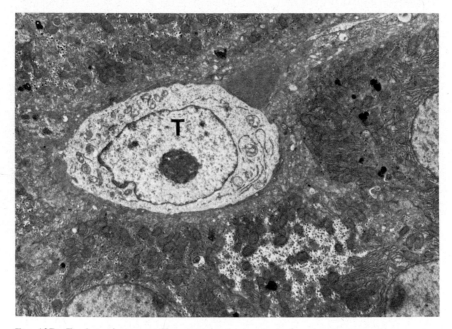

FIG. 12D. For legend *see* page 41

indicated that procedures as diverse as trauma, reticuloendothelial blockade and administration of dextran or high fat diets enhanced the growth of intrahepatic tumour without any increased local trapping of ^{51}-Cr-labelled tumour cells. Transaminase levels were often increased by these manoeuvres but the underlying changes were not clarified.

(4) Studies on hepatic metastases derived from a subcutaneously implanted lymphoma in hamsters indicated that treatment with a non-ionic detergent ("Triton WR 1339") enhanced intrahepatic tumour growth by producing changes in *host* rather than tumour tissues (Carter *et al.*, 1971; Carter and Cotmore, 1973; Cotmore and Carter, 1973—*see* Fig. 12). Pronounced morphological and biochemical alterations were seen in the liver lysosomes. It is interesting that the effects of this surfactant were not reproduced with other hamster tumours nor with a transplantable squamous carcinoma of the skin in rats (Pimm and Baldwin, 1975).

(5) A variant of most studies on "soil" factors is provided by the work of Pilgrim (1969) with a transplanted lymphoma in C3H mice that metastasised exclusively to the spleen. A comparison of growth of tumour injected directly into the preferred site (spleen) and a non-preferred site (kidney) suggested a differential rate of cell loss with greater migration from the non-preferred site.

(6) The work of Nicolson and his colleagues, assessing the organ specificity of tumour metastases by means of an *in vitro* cell adhesion technique (*see* Nicolson and Winkelhake, 1975; Winkelhake and Nicolson, 1976; Nicolson *et al.*, 1976) was discussed earlier in this chapter. The quantitative adhesion assays that have been devised measure both the rate and degree of attachment of tumour cells to monolayer substrates, and they provide a valuable method for analysing organ specificity both in terms of the attributes of the tissue and the tumour cell—the "soil" and the "seed".

4. Trauma

The tendency for metastases to develop preferentially at sites of trauma has long been familiar. Ludarsch in 1912 described the localization of tumour round wooden splinters implanted into the livers of mice, and Jones and Rous recorded in 1914 the enhanced growth of tumour cells injected intraperitoneally into mice pre-treated with intraperitoneal kieselguhr. This general association was confirmed by Fisher *et al.* (1967) who injected Walker tumour cells into the aorta of rats whose hind limbs had previously been traumatized by crush injuries, surgical incisions or by intramuscular

injections of turpentine. Consistently more tumours developed in
traumatized than in untraumatized limbs, with maximal effects in
animals with chemical damage inflicted by turpentine. The most
likely explanation for these findings is the local stimulus for tumour
growth provided by vascular proliferation, but it should be noted that
local trauma can potentiate tumour growth in several other ways—
notably by damaging vascular endothelium and by activating the
clotting mechanism.

5. Irradiation

Much attention has been paid to recent clinical and experimental
studies which indicate that metastasis in certain sites may be
enhanced by previous local irradiation—*see also Chapter III*. In
experimental animals, increased numbers of deposits, developing
from various intravenously injected tumour cells, have been described after local irradiation of the lungs (Fisher and Fisher, 1962;
Van den Brenk *et al.*, 1973; Withers and Milas, 1973) and the liver
and kidneys (Fisher and Fisher, 1969; Van den Brenk and Kelly,
1973). This increased incidence occurred only in the days immediately following irradiation—a time which seems too early to
invoke immunosuppressive effects. Furthermore, the doses of
irradiation used were generally too small for any such effects to be
produced. Studies with ^{51}Cr-labelled fibrosarcoma cells reported by
Withers and Milas (1973) suggested increased retention within the
pulmonary vasculature. Changes in pulmonary vessels or pulmonary
blood flow were not described in this account and the nature of the
radiation-induced changes which are temporarily conducive to the
establishment and growth of tumour deposits is unclear. It should be
noted that prior irradiation of the subcutaneous tissues is associated
with *impaired* growth of tumour subsequently implanted into the
treated area (Hewitt and Blake, 1968). This so-called "Tumour Bed
Effect" has long been known but its cause is obscure; defective
vascularization seems the most obvious possibility.

The clinical implications are particularly controversial (*see also
Chapter III*). In the case of breast cancer, for example, some workers
claim an increased incidence of metastases in the ipsilateral lung and
skin which fall into the treatment field. Patients with breast cancer
who receive post-operative radiotherapy tend to develop a circulating
lymphopenia (Meyer, 1970) which involves mainly T cells (Stjernswärd *et al.*, 1972). Survival in this irradiated group of breast cancer
patients now appears to be significantly decreased (Stjernswärd,

1974) though the extent and localization of their metastatic disease has not been reported.

6. Inflammatory responses

The possible interaction of the inflammatory response with metastasising tumour has received little attention. The point at which any such interaction might be most relevant is during the early extravascular phase of tumour growth (*see* Section VI). Most of the small amount of evidence available tends to suggest that a local inflammatory response may *facilitate* the establishment of metastatic tumour. The response may be initiated or augmented by release of pharmacological mediators such as prostaglandins by tumour cells or by host elements. Large doses of anti-inflammatory corticosteroids reduce the establishment, growth and spread of injected Yoshida and Walker cell lines in rats (Van den Brenk et al., 1974); other (non-corticosteroid) anti-inflammatory agents were shown to exert a similar effect. The components of the inflammatory response which potentiate tumour growth are unclear but the local development of vascular granulation tissue is likely to be important. Recent studies on graft-*versus*-host reactions, suggesting that immunocompetent lymphocytes may induce local angiogenesis, are of particular interest in this context (Sidky and Auerbach, 1975). In man, tumour cells have been shown to persist in skin windows despite a brisk inflammatory response (Brennan, 1968). On the other hand, a massive local infection such as an empyema may impair, or actually prove inimical to, tumour growth. More clinical and experimental studies on inflammation and growth of tumour cells are needed and, in the particular context of localization of metastatic tumour, it should be borne in mind that inflammatory responses may vary on a regional basis and may be impaired by immunosuppression.

7. Immunological responses

The distribution of circulating tumour cells may in part be determined by the immunological status of the host. Weiss et al. (1974a) compared the distribution of two species of ^{125}I-UDR-labelled tumour cells—from the Gardner lymphosarcoma and from a methylcholanthrene-induced fibrosarcoma—one hour after intravenous injection into normal C3H mice, into tumour-bearing mice and into hyperimmunized mice. The patterns of distribution varied for the two tumours and also according to the recipients' immune status. In normal mice, most fibrosarcoma cells ($>90\%$) localized in the lungs; in immunized and tumour-bearing animals the proportion of intrapulmonary cells fell and the fraction of tumour cells in the liver, lymphoid tissues and kidney was increased. Lymphosarcoma cells in normal mice were distributed in the lungs and the liver but (in contrast to the previous findings) the proportion of pulmonary tumour cells rose in the sensitized groups. On the other hand, Weston et al. (1974), using an allogeneic system, found that ^{125}I-IUDR-labelled EL$_4$ lymphoma cells showed no significant differences in their patterns of distribution when injected intravenously into normal and T-cell deficient CBA mice—even though the T cell-deficient animals all died early with massive visceral deposits while the normal mice died after a long interval with small amounts of tumour confined to soft tissues; some normal animals remained free of tumour. T cell-deficient mice reconstituted with a syngeneic thymus graft behaved like normal animals—see Chapter II.

There is a little evidence to suggest that the immune response to tumours may vary in effectiveness in different anatomical regions. Vaage et al. (1971) immunized C3H mice with a syngeneic methylcholanthrene-induced fibrosarcoma and examined the effects of immune status on the growth of a tumour challenge given at one of four sites: subcutaneous tissues, peritoneal cavity, lungs (via tail vein) and liver (via hepatic portal bein). Resistance in the liver and lungs was more marked than in the subcutaneous tissues or peritoneal cavity; the degree of resistance in each site varied according to the mode of immunization; and a combination of immunization and immunotherapy (killed tumour cells given subcutaneously after challenge) yielded more protection than immunization alone. Using a rather different approach, Alexander et al. (1973) have shown that DBA2 mice with growing tumour (the L5178Y lymphoma) implanted in their flanks will reject challenges of the same tumour injected into the peritoneal cavity. They adduced evidence that the local intraperitoneal immunity may be mediated by macrophages.

Procedures such as treatment with antilymphocyte serum (ALS) or T cell deprivation may enhance metastatic growth (Deodhar and Crile, 1969; Gershon and Carter, 1970), and Weston and her colleagues (1974) showed that T-cell deprivation affected not only the incidence but also the amount and anatomical distribution of metastatic tumour derived from a subcutaneous allograft of the EL4 lymphoma. The effects of immunosuppression on metastasis are discussed in more detail in Chapter VI but it should be noted that some immunosuppressive regimes have not resulted in uniformly enhanced metastatic growth (Boeryd and Suurküla, 1973; Suurküla and Boeryd, 1974).

8. The intrinsic properties of the tumour cells

The extent to which the intrinsic characteristics of disseminating tumour cells may determine their final location in the body is obscure. Membrane properties have been implicated in the adhesion of tumour cells to endothelium (*see* p. 26 *et seq.*) and, in the extravascular compartment, in their locomotion and ability to establish cell-to-cell contacts, either with other tumour cells or with inflammatory and immune cells (Weiss, 1967, 1976). Experimental demonstration of such fundamental properties of tumour cells is, however, proving difficult. Treatment of Walker carcinosarcoma cells with neuraminidase, sufficient to drop their surface charge by about 30%, produced no significant alteration in their distribution at 5 and 60 minutes after intravenous injection in rats (Weiss *et al.*, 1974b). This finding contrasts with the profound alteration in "homing" which occurs when thoracic duct lymphocytes are exposed to neuraminidase. Heparin appears, *inter alia*, to alter the distribution of tumour cells both within the vascular compartment (Hagmar and Noorby, 1970; Hagmar, 1972b) and between the vascular and lymphatic circuits (Hilgard *et al.*, 1972). Distribution of intravascular tumour cells may also be effected by trypsin (Hagmar and Norrby, 1973) and by dextran (Hagmar, 1972b) but the underlying mechanisms, as with heparin, are complex and obscure. The *in vitro* studies of homotypic and heterotypic tumour cell adhesion reported by Nicolson and his colleagues were discussed at the beginning of this chapter.

One final comment may be made on a general clinical aspect of the localization of metastatic tumour. The recognized patterns of metastasis are not immutable, and it is becoming clear that established patterns may change, sometimes as a result of longer survival times or perhaps as a consequence of treatment. More patients with cancers of the head and neck are found to have metastases in sites below the clavicle such as mediastinal lymph nodes, lungs, liver or bone (Probert *et al.*, 1974). The incidence of extrapulmonary metastases in osteosarcoma appears to be higher than was previously recognized (Jeffree *et al.*, 1975). Lastly, changes in the distribution of metastases, associated with treatment, were proposed several years ago in patients with breast cancer treated with adrenal corticosteroids (Iversen and Hjort, 1958; Sherlock and Hartmann, 1962); the potential capacity for elaborate modern drug schedules to modify the amount and distribution of metastatic tumour is likely to be considerable.

REFERENCES

Abe, R. and Taneichi, N. (1972). *Arch. Surg.* **104**, 95–98.
Alexander, P., Evans, R. and Mikulska, Z. B. (1973). *In* "Chemotherapy of Cancer Dissemination and Metastasis" (S. Garattini and G. Franchi, eds.), pp. 177–185. Raven Press, New York.
Atherton, A. (1975). *Europ. J. Cancer*, **11**, 383–388.
Atherton, A. and Born, G. V. R. (1972). *J. Physiol.* **222**, 447–474.
Atherton, A. and Born, G. V. R. (1973). *J. Physiol.* **233**, 157–165.
Baserga, R., Kisieleski, W. E. and Halvorsen, K. (1960). *Cancer Res.* **20**, 910–917.
Bennett, A., McDonald, A. M., Simpson, J. S. and Stamford, I. F. (1975). *Lancet*, i, 1218–1220.
Berge, T. (1974). *Acta path. microbiol. scand.* (*A*) **82**, 499–506.
Boeryd, B. and Suurküla, M. (1973). *Int. J. Cancer* **12**, 722–727.
Bosmann, H. B., Bieber, G. F., Brown, A. E., Case, K. R., Gerstein, D. M., Kimmerer, T. W. and Lione, A. (1973). *Nature, Lond.* **246**, 487–489.
Brem, S., Brem, H., Folkman, J., Finkelstein, D. and Patz, A. (1976). *Cancer Res.* **36**, 2807–2812.
Brem, H. and Folkman, J. (1975). *J. exp. Med.* **141**, 427–439.
Brennan, M. J. (1968). *In* "The Proliferation and Spread of Neoplastic Cells". 21st Annual Symposium on Fundamental Cancer Research, 1967, pp. 607–613. University of Texas, M.D. Anderson Hospital and Tumor Institute at Houston, Texas. Williams and Wilkins, Baltimore.
Brown, J. M. (1973). *Cancer Res.* **33**, 1217–1224.
Burn, J. I. (1968). *Ann. R. Coll. Surg. Engl.* **42**, 93–113.
Butler, T. P. and Gullino, P. M. (1975). *Cancer Res.* **35**, 512–516.
Cameron, G. R. (1954). *Brit. med. J.* **1**, 347–352.
Candar, Z., Ritchie, A. C., Hopkirk, J. F. and Long, R. C. (1962). *Surg. Gynec. Obstet.* **115**, 291–294.
Carr, I., McGinty, F. and Norris, P. (1976). *J. Path.* **118**, 91–99.
Carter, R. L. and Gershon, R. K. (1966). *Amer. J. Path.* **49**, 637–655.
Carter, R. L. and Gershon, R. K. (1967). *Amer. J. Path.* **50**, 203–217.
Carter, R. L., Birbeck, M. S. C. and Stock, J. A. (1971). *Int. J. Cancer* **7**, 34–49.
Carter, R. L. and Cotmore, S. F. (1973). *In* "Chemotherapy of Cancer Dissemination and Metastasis" (S. Garattini and G. Franchi, eds.), pp. 325–339. Raven Press, New York.
Carter, R. L. (1975a). *In* "Host Defence in Breast Cancer" (B. A. Stoll, ed.), pp. 6–35. Heinemann Medical Books, London.
Carter, R. L. (1975b). *In* "Biology of Cancer" (E. J. Ambrose and F. J. C. Roe, eds.), pp. 74–95, 2nd edn. Ellis Horwood, Chichester.
Cater, D. B., Adair, H. M. and Grove, C. A. (1966). *Brit. J. Cancer* **20**, 504–516.
Cater, D. B. and Taylor, C. R. (1966). *Brit. J. Cancer*, **20**, 517–525.
Charbit, A., Malaise, E. P. and Tubiana, M. (1971). *Europ. J. Cancer*, **7**, 307–315.
Chew, E. C., Josephson, R. L. and Wallace, A. C. (1976). *In* "Fundamental Aspects of Metastasis" (L. Weiss, ed.), pp. 121–150. North-Holland Publishing Company, Amsterdam-Oxford.
Coates, G., Bush, R. S. and Aspin, N. (1973). *Radiology*, **107**, 577–583.

Coman, D. R. (1953). *Cancer Res.* **13**, 397–404.
Coman, D. R. and de Long, R. P. (1951). *Cancer, N. Y.* **14**, 610–618.
Conzelman, G. M. and Springer, K. (1969). *Cancer Chemotherapy Rep. Part 1*, **53**, 105–113.
Cotmore, S. F. and Carter, R. L. (1973). *Int. J. Cancer*, **11**, 725–738.
Crile, G., Jr. (1966). *Ann. Surg.* **163**, 267–271.
Crile, G., Jr., Isbister, W. and Deodhar, S. D. (1971). *Cancer, Philad.* **28**, 655–656.
Davidsohn, I. (1972). *Amer. J. clin. Path.* **57**, 715–730.
Deodhar, S. D. and Crile, G., Jr. (1969). *Cancer Res.* **29**, 776–779.
Dowsett, M., Eastman, A. R., Easty, D. M., Easty, G. C., Powles, T. J. and Neville, A. M. (1976). *Nature, Lond.* **263**, 72–74.
Drury, R. A. B., Palmer, P. H. and Highman, W. J. (1964). *J. clin. Path.* **17**, 448–457.
Edwards, M. H., Baum, M. and Magarey, C. J. (1972). *Brit. J. Surg.* **59**, 776–779.
Elias, E. G., Sepulveda, F. and Mink, I. B. (1973). *J. Surg. Oncol.* **5**, 189.
Engesett, A. (1966). *Progr. exp. Tumor Res.* **8**, 225–270.
Engzell, U., Rubio, C., Tjernberg, B. and Zajicek, J. (1968). *Europ. J. Cancer*, **4**, 305–312.
Everson, T. C. and Cole, W. H. (1966). "Spontaneous Regression of Cancer". Saunders, Philadelphia and London.
Fastaia, J. and Dumont, A. E. (1976). *J. Natl. Cancer Inst.*, **56**, 547–550.
Feldman, G. B. (1975). *Cancer Res.* **35**, 325–332.
Feldman, G. B. and Knapp, R. C. (1974). *Amer. J. Obstet. Gynec.* **119**, 991–994.
Fidler, I. J. (1970). *J. Natl. Cancer Inst.*, **45**, 773–782.
Fidler, I. J. (1973a). *Nature New Biol.* **242**, 148–149.
Fidler, I. J. (1973b). *Europ. J. Cancer*, **9**, 223–227.
Fidler, I. J. (1975). *Cancer Res.* **35**, 218–224.
Fidler, I. J. (1976). *In* "Cancer: A Comprehensive Treatise", Vol. 4 (F. F. Becker, ed.), pp. 101–131. Plenum Press, New York and London.
Fisch, U. (1970). *In* "Progress in Clinical Cancer", Vol. IV (I. Ariel, ed.). Grune and Stratton, New York.
Fisher, B. and Fisher, E. R. (1959). *Ann. Surg.* **150**, 731–734.
Fisher, B. and Fisher, E. R. (1962). *Surg. Clin. N. Amer.* **42**, 335–339.
Fisher, B. and Fisher, E. R. (1966). *Science*, **152**, 1397–1398.
Fisher, B. and Fisher, E. R. (1967a). *Cancer, Philad.* **20**, 1907 and 1914–1919.
Fisher, B. and Fisher, E. R. (1967b). *Cancer Res.* **27**, 412 120.
Fisher, B., Fisher, E. R. and Feduska, N. (1967). *Cancer, Philad.* **20**, 23–30.
Fisher, B. and Fisher, E. R. (1968). *In* "The Proliferation and Spread of Neoplastic Cells". 21st Annual Symposium on Fundamental Cancer Research, 1967, pp. 555–582. University of Texas, M.D. Anderson Hospital and Tumor Institute at Houston, Texas. Williams and Wilkins, Baltimore.
Fisher, E. R. and Fisher, B. (1969). *Cancer Res.* **24**, 39–55.
Fisher, E. R., Gregorio, R. M., Redmond, C., Kim, W. S. and Fisher, B. (1976). *Amer. J. clin. Path.* **65**, 439–444.
Folkman, J. (1974). *Adv. Cancer Res.* **19**, 331–358.
Folkman, J. (1975). *Ann. intern. Med.* **82**, 96–100.
Futtrell, J. W. and Pories, W. J. (1975). *Surg. Gynec. Obstet.* **140**, 273–278.
Gasic, G. J., Gasic, T. B. and Stewart, C. E. (1968). *Proc. Nat. Acad. Sci., Wash.* **61**, 46–52.
Gershon, R. K., Carter, R. L. and Kondo, K. (1967). *Nature, Lond.* **213**, 674–676.
Gershon, R. K., Carter, R. L. and Kondo, K. (1968). *Science*, **159**, 646–648.

Gershon, R. K. and Carter, R. L. (1970). *Nature, Lond.* **226**, 368–370.

Gimbrone, M. A., Jr., Leapman, S. B., Cotran, R. S. and Folkman, J. (1972). *J. exp. Med.*, **136**, 261–276.

Gimbrone, M. A., Leapman, S. B., Cotran, R. S. and Folkman, J. (1973). *J. Natl. Cancer Inst.* **50**, 219–225.

Griffiths, J. D. and Salsbury, A. J. (1965). "Circulating Cancer Cells". C. C. Thomas, Springfield, Illinois.

Griffiths, J. D., McKinna, J. A., Rowbotham, H. D., Tsolakidis, P. and Salsbury, A. J. (1973). *Cancer, Philad.* **31**, 226–236.

Hagmar, B. (1970). *Acta path. microbiol. scand.* (*A*), **78**, 131–142.

Hagmar, B. (1972a). *Europ. J. Cancer*, **8**, 17–28.

Hagmar, B. (1972b). *Acta path. microbiol. scand.* (*A*), **80**, 357–366.

Hagmar, B. and Norrby, K. (1970). *Int. J. Cancer*, **5**, 72–84.

Hagmar, B. and Norrby, K. (1973). *Int. J. Cancer*, **11**, 663–675.

Hall, J. G. (1969). *New Engl. J. Med.* **281**, 720–722.

Harris, M., Jenkins, M. V., Bennet, A. and Wills, M. R. (1973). *Nature, Lond.* **245**, 213–215.

Herman, P. G., Ohba, S. and Mellins, H. Z. (1969). *Radiology*, **92**, 1073–1080.

Herman, P. G., Yamamoto, I. and Mellins, H. Z. (1972). *J. exp. Med.* **136**, 697–714.

Hewitt, H. B. and Blake, E. R. (1968). *Brit. J. Cancer*, **22**, 808–824.

Hilgard, P., Beyerle, L., Hohage, R., Hiemeyer, V. and Kübler, M. (1972). *Europ. J. Cancer*, **8**, 347–352.

Hilgard, P. (1973). *Brit. J. Cancer*, **28**, 429–435.

Hirabayashi, K. and Graham, J. (1970). *Amer. J. Obstet. Gynec.* **106**, 492–497.

Hirano, A. and Zimmerman, H. M. (1972). *Lab. Invest.* **26**, 465–468.

Holyoke, E. D., Frank, A. L. and Weiss, L. (1972). *Int. J. Cancer*, **9**, 258–263.

Iversen, H-G. and Hjort, G. H. (1958). *Acta path. microbiol. scand.* **44**, 205–212.

Jeffree, G. M., Price, C. H. G. and Sissons, H. A. (1975). *Brit. J. Cancer*, **32**, 87–107.

Jones, D. S., Wallace, A. C. and Fraser, E. E. (1971). *J. Natl. Cancer Inst.* **46**, 493–504.

Kim, U. (1966). *Cancer Res.* **26**, 461–463.

Kim, U. (1970). *Science*, **167**, 72.

Kim, U., Baumler, A., Carruthers, C. and Bielar, K. (1975). *Proc. Natl. Acad. Sci. U.S.A.* **72**, 1012–1016.

Kinsey, D. L. (1960). *Cancer*, **13**, 674–676.

Langer, R., Brem, H., Falterman, K., Klein, W. and Folkman, J. (1976). *Science*, **193**, 70–72.

Lill, P. H., Norris, H. J., Rubenstone, A. I., Chang-Lo, M. and Davidsohn, I. (1976). *Amer. J. clin. Path.* **66**, 767–774.

Liotta, L. A., Kleinerman, J. and Saidel, G. M. (1974). *Cancer Res.* **34**, 997–1004.

Liotta, L. A., Kleinerman, J. and Saidel, G. M. (1976). *Cancer Res.* **36**, 889–894.

de Long, R. P. and Coman, D. R. (1950). *Cancer Res.* **10**, 513–515.

Lucké, B., Breedis, C., Woo, Z. P., Bewick, L. and Nowell, P. (1952). *Cancer Res.*, **12**, 734–739.

Ludatscher, R. M., Luse, S. A. and Suntzeff, V. (1967). *Cancer Res.* **27**, 1939–1952.

Ludwig, J. and Titus, J. L. (1967). *Archs. Path.* **84**, 304–311.

Luk, S. C., Nopajaroonsri, C. and Simon, G. T. (1973). *Clin. Invest.* **29**, 258.

Malmgren, R. A. (1968). *In* "The Proliferation and Spread of Neoplastic Cells". 21st Annual Symposium on Fundamental Cancer Research, 1967, pp. 481–494. University of Texas, M.D. Anderson Hospital and Tumor Institute at Houston, Texas. Williams and Wilkins, Baltimore.

Meyer, K. K. (1970). *Arch. Surg.* **101**, 114–121.
Meyers, M. A. (1973). *Amer. J. Roentgenol.* **119**, 198–206.
Michaels, L. (1964). *Lancet*, ii, 832–835.
Mundy, G. R., Luben, R. A., Raisz, L. G., Oppenheim, J. J. and Buell, D. N. (1974a). *New Engl. J. Med.* **290**, 867–871.
Mundy, G. R., Raisz, L. G., Cooper, R. A., Schechter, G. P. and Salmon, S. E. (1974b). *New Engl. J. Med.* **291**, 1041–1046.
Nicolson, G. L. and Winkelhake, J. L. (1975). *Nature, Lond.* **255**, 230–232.
Nicolson, G. L., Winkelhake, J. L. and Nussey, C. (1976). *In* "Fundamental Aspects of Metastasis" (L. Weiss, ed.), pp. 291–303. North-Holland Publishing Company, Amsterdam-Oxford.
Oikawa, M., Milne, E. N. C., Whitmore, E., Gilday, E. and Oliver, C. (1975). *Cancer, Philad.* **35**, 385–398.
Papadimitriou, J. M. and Woods, A. E. (1975). *J. Path.* **116**, 65–72.
Peters, L. J. (1975). *Br. J. Cancer*, **32**, 355–365.
Pilgrim, H. I. (1969). *Cancer Res.* **29**, 1200–1205.
Pimm, M. V. and Baldwin, R. W. (1975). *Brit. J. Cancer*, **31**, 62–67.
Plenk, H. P., Sorenson, F. M. and Eichwald, E. J. (1954). *Cancer Res.* **14**, 580–581.
Powles, T. J., Clark, S. A., Easty, D. M., Easty, G. C. and Neville, A. M. (1973). *Brit. J. Cancer*, **28**, 316–321.
Powles, T. J., Dowsett, M., Easty, G. C., Easty, D. M. and Neville, A. M. (1976). *Lancet*, i, 608–610.
Pressman, J. J., Burtz, M. V. and Shafer, L. (1964). *Surg. Gynec. Obstet.* **119**, 984–990.
Pressman, J. J., Simon, M. B., Hand, K. and Miller, J. (1962). *Surg. Gynec. Obst.* **115**, 207–214.
Probert, J. C., Thompson, R. W. and Bagshaw, M. A. (1974). *Cancer, Philad.* **33**, 127–133.
Rodin, A. E., Larsen, D. L. and Roberts, D. K. (1967). *Cancer, Philad.* **20**, 1772–1779.
Romsdahl, M. D., Chu, E. W., Hume, R. and Smith, R. R. (1961). *Cancer, Philad.* **14**, 883–888.
Ryan, J. J., Ketcham, A. S. and Wexler, H. (1968). *Ann. Surg.* **168**, 163–168.
Salsbury, A. J., Burrage, K. and Hellman, K. (1974). *Cancer Res.* **34**, 843–849.
Salsbury, A. J. (1975). *Cancer Treat. Rev.* **2**, 55–72.
Sato, H. and Suzuki, M. (1972). *In* "Proc. International Symposium on Atherogenesis and Thrombogenesis", pp. 168–176. Excerpta Medica, Amsterdam.
Schabell, F. M. (1975). *Cancer, Philad.* **35**, 15–24.
Le Serve, A. W. and Hellmann, K. (1972). *Brit. med. J.*, **1**, 597–601.
Sherlock, P. and Hartmann, W. H. (1962). *J. Am. med. Assn.* **181**, 313–317.
Sherman, J. O. and O'Brien, P. H. (1967). *Cancer, Philad.* **20**, 1851–1858.
Shivas, A. A. and Finlayson, N. D. C. (1965). *Brit. J. Cancer*, **19**, 486–489.
Sidky, Y. A. and Auerbach, R. (1975). *J. exp. Med.* **141**, 1084–1100
Slack, N. H. and Bross, I. D. J. (1975). *Brit. J. Cancer*, **32**, 78–86.
Smithers, D. W. (1969). *Lancet*, ii, 949–952.
Söderström, N. and Norberg, B. (1974). *Acta path. microbiol. scand. (A)*, **82**, 71–79.
Stjernswärd, J., Jondal, M., Vánky, F., Wigzell, H. and Sealy, R. (1972). *Lancet*, i, 1352–1356.
Stjernswärd, J. (1974). *Lancet*, ii, 1285–1286.

Stoker, T. A. M. (1969). *Brit. J. Cancer*, **23**, 132 and 136–140.

Sugarbaker, E. V., Ketcham, A. S. and Cohen, A. M. (1971). *Cancer, Philad.* **28**, 545–552.

Suurküla, M. and Boeryd, B. (1974). *Int. J. Cancer*, **14**, 633–641.

Tannock, I. F. (1970). *Cancer Res.* **30**, 2470–2476.

Tannock, I. F. and Hayashi, S. (1972). *Cancer Res.* **32**, 77–82.

Taptiklis, N. (1968). *Europ. J. Cancer*, **4**, 59–66.

Taptiklis, N. (1969). *Europ. J. Cancer*, **5**, 445–457.

Tashjian, A. H., Voelkel, E. F., Goldhaber, P. and Levine, L. (1974). *Fed. Proc.* **33**, 81–86.

Treidman, L. and McNeer, G. (1963). *Ann. N. Y. Acad. Sci.* **100**, 123–130.

Underwood, J. C. E. and Carr, I. (1972). *J. Path.* **107**, 157–166.

Vaage, J., Chen, K. and Merrick, S. (1971). *Cancer Res.* **31**, 496–500.

Van den Brenk, H. A. S., Burch, W. M., Orton, C. and Sharpington, C. (1973). *Brit. J. Cancer*, **27**, 291–306.

Van den Brenk, H. A. S. and Kelly, H. (1973). *Brit. J. Cancer*, **28**, 349–353.

Van den Brenk, H. A. S., Kelly, H. and Orton, C. (1974). *Brit. J. Cancer*, **29**, 365–372.

Van den Brenk, H. A. S., Burch, W. M., Kelly, H. and Orton, C. (1975). *Brit. J. Cancer*, **31**, 46–61.

Warren, B. A. (1970). *Brit. J. exp. Path.* **51**, 570–580.

Warren, B. A. and Vales, O. (1972). *Brit. J. exp. Path.* **53**, 301–313.

Weiss, L. (1967). "The Cell Periphery, Metastasis and Other Contact Phenomena". North Holland, Amsterdam.

Weiss, L. (1973). *In* "Chemotherapy of Cancer Dissemination and Metastasis" (S. Garattini and G. Franchi, eds.), pp. 19–30. Raven Press, New York.

Weiss, L., Glaves, D. and Waite, D. A. (1974a). *Int. J. Cancer*, **13**, 850–862.

Weiss, L., Fisher, B. and Fisher, E. R. (1974b). *Cancer, Philad.* **34**, 680–683.

Weiss, L. (1976) (ed.). "Fundamental Aspects of Metastasis". North-Holland Publishing Company, Amsterdam-Oxford.

Weston, B. J., Carter, R. L., Easty, G. C., Connell, D. I. and Davies, A. J. S. (1974). *Int. J. Cancer*, **14**, 176–185.

Wexler, H., Ryan, J. J. and Ketcham, A. S. (1969). *Cancer, Philad.* **23**, 946–951.

Wilder, R. J. (1956). *J. Mt. Sinai Hosp.* **23**, 728.

Willis, R. A. (1973). "Spread of Tumours in the Human Body". 3rd edn. Butterworths, London.

Winkelhake, J. L. and Nicolson, G. L. (1976). *J. Natl. Cancer Inst.* **56**, 285–291.

Withers, H. R. and Milas, L. (1973). *Cancer Res.* **33**, 1931–1936.

Wood, P. and Carr, I. (1974). *J. Path.* **114**, 85–88.

Wood, S., Jr. (1958). *Archs. Path.* **66**, 550–568.

Wood, S., Jr. (1971). *In* "Pathobiology Annual", Vol. 1 (H. L. Ioachim, ed.), pp. 281–308. Butterworths, London.

Yoffey, J. M. and Courtice, F. C. (1970). "Lymphatics, Lymph and the Lymphomyeloid Complex". Academic Press, New York and London.

Zeidman, I. (1961). *Cancer Res.* **21**, 38–39.

Zeidman, I. and Buss, J. M. (1952). *Cancer Res.* **12**, 731–733.

Zeidman, I. and Buss, J. M. (1954). *Cancer Res.* **14**, 403–405.

Chapter II

Some Lymphoreticular Reactions and the Metastatic Process

R. L. CARTER

Institute of Cancer Research and Royal Marsden Hospital, Sutton, Surrey, England

I. Introduction

There is scattered evidence from clinical and experimental sources which indicates that immune reactions may affect the metastatic growth of certain tumours; but it is difficult to isolate components of the immune response which impinge *specifically* on the metastatic process as opposed to other facets of tumour growth. The problem is encountered equally in circumstances where immune responses seem to be associated with a reduced tendency to metastatic spread, and where the impairment or absence of any such immune response is accompanied by an increased incidence of metastases. There are, however, four particular stages in the metastatic process (cf. Chapter I) where immune responses may act:

(1) The initial phases of release of tumour cells from the primary tumour.
(2) Circulating tumour cells, including patterns of early arrest.
(3) The initial phases of extravascular growth of micrometastases.
(4) Early responses in regional lymph nodes.

Many of these aspects are discussed in *Chapter VI*, and the present account deals mainly with lymphoreticular reactions at two sites— the primary tumour and the regional lymph nodes.

II. Lymphoreticular Changes Associated with Primary Tumours

Certain human tumours—notably some mammary carcinomas, seminomas, choriocarcinomas and melanomas—are surrounded by a dense infiltrate of macrophages, lymphocytes and plasma cells. An example of a heavily infiltrated medullary carcinoma of the breast is shown in Fig. 1. Such tumours carry a better prognosis than otherwise similar neoplasms where a local host cell infiltrate is scanty or absent. Infiltrated tumours appear, *inter alia*, less likely to metastasise though it seems too simple to equate their generally more favourable outcome solely with reduced metastatic spread.

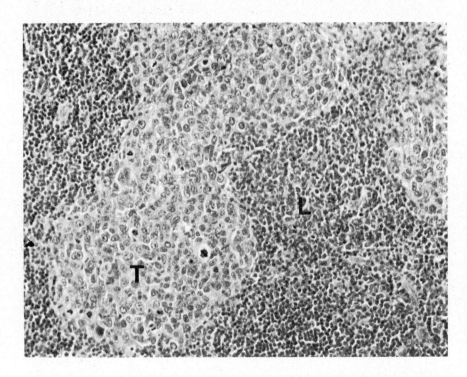

FIG. 1. Medullary carcinoma of breast from 41-year-old woman. Poorly differentiated tumour cells (T) are enclosed by a dense infiltrate of lymphoid cells (L). Treated by radical mastectomy. Patient remains disease-free after 20 years

The significance of these host cell infiltrates *in human tumours* is ill-understood (Carr and Underwood, 1974; Underwood, 1974). Some of the cellular components are difficult to characterize by conventional morphology, and histochemistry, electron microscopy and surface markers are required for accurate identification of the various cell types (Underwood and Carr, 1972; Underwood, 1974; Roubin *et al.*, 1975). The origin and function of some of the large non-phagocytic mononuclear cells which have recently been described in such infiltrates is unknown. The overall appearance of the infiltrates does not resemble a typical homograft rejection, nor a delayed hypersensitivity-type reaction such as the kind induced when tumours are treated with local injections of BCG. Few authors have seen any morphological evidence of confrontation between tumour cells and infiltrating host cells in the light or electron microscope.

Host cell infiltrates in tumours are technically easier to study *in experimental animals* (Kerbel and Davies, 1974; Kerbel *et al.*, 1975; Wood and Gillespie, 1975). Using F_c membrane receptors as host cell markers, these authors have shown that several epithelial and mesenchymal tissues in rats and mice contain a variable but often surprisingly high proportion (5–61%) of F_c-bearing cells. The F_c-positive cells are a heterogeneous group. Phagocytic macrophages predominate but activated T cells are also present and probably K cells, B cells and neutrophils as well (cf. Kerbel and Davies, 1974). Apart from certain lymphomas and leukaemias, it appears that neoplastic cells hardly ever carry F_c receptors on their surfaces and, at the present time, it is reasonable to conclude that F_c receptor-bearing cells in tumours are predominantly or exclusively of host origin.

The intensity of host cell infiltration in some of these tumours is clearly more extensive than might have been guessed, and the presence of this large host component must now be taken into account in studies of the cell biology of tumours. The specific relevance of host cell infiltrates to metastasis is not clear, but interesting results have been reported by Wood and Gillespie (1975) who prepared suspensions of various murine tumours, removed the associated macrophages by adherence to plastic Petri dishes and then injected the tumour cells subcutaneously into syngeneic recipients. Compared to control animals receiving "untreated" tumour cell inocula, the test mice developed pulmonary and/or lymph node metastases, and their survival times were shortened. The content of F_c-containing cells in the metastatic deposits was not determined. These results bear out previous observations by Eccles and

Alexander (1974; *see also* Alexander, 1976) in syngeneic 3,4-benzopyrene-induced fibrosarcomas in rats. Here, an inverse correlation was noted between the macrophage level of the tumours and their proclivity to metastasise; the rats had previously been rendered T cell deficient either by chronic thoracic duct drainage or by thymectomy combined with whole body irradiation. In separate experiments with the MC3 sarcoma in hooded rats, Eccles and Alexander tested the effects of non-specific stimulation with BCG prior to tumour inoculation; they reported a moderate increase in macrophage infiltration in the tumours and a small decline in the incidence of spontaneous metastases. Earlier morphological studies with two hamster lymphomas (Gershon *et al.*, 1967a; Birbeck and Carter, 1972; *see also* p. 65) are relevant here as well: large numbers of activated macrophages are regularly present in a non-metastasising lymphoma (NML) but scarce or absent in a morphologically similar lesion (ML) which invariably metastasises.

It is, however, important not to over-interpret the macrophage infiltrates found in tumours as they may accumulate for a variety of reasons. Some of the cells may be fulfilling simple scavenging functions, others may be "innocent bystanders". An unknown proportion may be involved in antitumour immune reactions, operating either in collaboration with other immune cells or as specifically "armed" antitumour macrophages; but this remains a controversial field and results, for example, from *in vitro* cytotoxicity of macrophages separated from tumours, are conflicting (Alexander, 1976). It should also be noted that there is evidence that the presence of an implanted tumour seems to *depress* the accumulation of macrophages at a distant inflammatory focus (Snyderman *et al.*, 1976). Lastly, it is emphasized that macrophages are the predominant, but not the exclusive, F_c-bearing host cell found in tumours. The role of lymphocytic infiltrates is illustrated by the studies of Weston and her colleagues (Weston *et al.*, 1972, 1974) with solid intradermal implants of the EL4 lymphoma, growing as an allograft in chimaeric CBA mice. There are two principal observations:

(1) A gross correlation was established between the accumulation of a local lymphocytic infiltrate and a temporary impairment in growth of the tumour graft, both coinciding with peak levels of T cell proliferation in the paracortex of the draining lymph nodes—*see also* p. 61.

(2) If the EL4 lymphoma was grafted into T cell-*deficient* mice, it

was not infiltrated by host cells and it metastasised in about 50% of animals.

III. Regional Lymph Nodes

Interpretation of reactive changes in lymph nodes draining poten-tially metastasising tumours has been aided by advances in know-ledge of the structure and function of the lymphoid tissues—notably in relation to the demarcation of T and B cell zones, and their different patterns of response. The morphological features of immune stimulation are similar in man and in laboratory animals, but certain general points of difference may be noted.

In *man*, opportunities to study truly normal lymph nodes are exceptional. Variations occur as a result of age, anatomical location, and the nature and extent of any underlying disease. Anatomical groups of lymph nodes comprise large numbers so that antigenic stimuli from a single focus impinge on many draining nodes. Some useful background information is, however, available in the autopsy study of axillary lymph nodes reported by Tsakraklides *et al.* (1975a). In *laboratory animals*, variables due to age and anatomical location can be standardized, normal nodes are readily available, the evolution of morphological responses may be followed over a time course, and comparisons made between events in local and more distal lymphoid structures. The numbers of nodes in a particular anatomical group is small. Whereas a mammary carcinoma in a woman provides a focus of chronic antigenic stimulation for 20 or 30 axillary nodes, the antigenic stimulus from a mammary carcinoma in a mouse falls on only 2 or 3 axillary nodes.

Morphological changes in uninvolved lymph nodes draining human tumours have been described in various contexts, notably in relation to carcinomas of the *breast* (Black *et al.*, 1953, 1955; Anastassiades and Pryce, 1966; Hamlin, 1968; Alderson *et al.*, 1971; Tsakraklides *et al.*, 1974), *stomach* (Black *et al.*, 1954, 1971), *cervix uteri* (Tsakraklides *et al.*, 1973), *colon and rectum* (Tsakraklides *et al.*, 1975b; Patt *et al.*, 1975), and *head and neck* (Bennett *et al.*, 1971; Berlinger *et al.*, 1976). The morphological changes are categorized in different ways by different authors. Tsakraklides and his colleagues use four terms—lymphocyte predominance, germinal centre pre-dominance, unstimulated and lymphocyte-depleted—which are simple and self-explanatory. As a very broad generalization, lymphocyte predominance in uninvolved nodes tends to be a favourable prognostic feature associated with the highest survival rates. Nodes which are inactive or show lymphocyte depletion tend to predominate in patients whose local nodes are beginning to be involved by metastatic disease and where survival rates are low. Germinal centre activation also appears more commonly when nodal spread has occurred.

Several discrepancies remain unresolved. In particular, the relevance of reactive changes in local lymph nodes is disputed in cancers of the head and neck (Bennett *et al.*, 1971; Berlinger *et al.*, 1976) and in colorectal malignancies (Tsakraklides *et al.*, 1975b; Patt *et al.*, 1975). There is also disagreement over the relative importance of lymphoreticular reactions in the vicinity of the primary tumour and in the regional nodes (*see* Hamlin, 1968; Alderson *et al.*, 1971; Turner and Berry, 1972) and in the ranking of the various morphological changes within the lymph nodes themselves. The implications of sinus histiocytosis are still disputed, and there are the more general problems of adequate sampling of large numbers of nodes from a surgical specimen and the continuing uncertainty over the nature of the stimuli which evoke the lymphoid responses—are they tumour-specific antigens and tumour-associated products, or is there an element of non-specific stimulation accruing from local infection, haemorrhage and necrosis?

A number of other approaches have been used to supplement lymph node morphology in human studies.

(1) Burtin *et al.* (1969) examined immunofluorescent staining in nodes draining mammary and other carcinomas. Immunoglobulins were abundant in histologically active nodes though some well-developed follicles did not contain stainable material. Immunoglobulins were still detectable in nodes partially replaced by metastatic tumour. IgA was the commonest immunoglobulin found, then IgM, then IgG. The predominance of (non-cytotoxic) IgA is curious and the authors suggested that it might represent a reaction to tumour products rather than to intact tumour cells (*vide supra*).

(2) Surface markers for T and B lymphocytes have been used by Tsakraklides *et al.* (1975c) to study the composition of axillary lymph nodes draining breast cancers. Increased proportions of T cells were found in lymphocyte predominant nodes; increased proportions of B cells were found in nodes showing germinal centre predominance, in nodes partly involved by metastases, and in nodes from older patients

(>60 years). The wider implications of these results are still to be assessed in mammary and other cancers but this approach is a potentially important one.

(3) Fisher *et al.* (1972) studied responses to phytohaemagglutinin (PHA) in cells from regional nodes and from the blood in patients with carcinomas of the breast and colon. Broadly similar results were obtained in both groups. Cells from almost all regional nodes responded to PHA, and responses were greater with cells from uninvolved nodes than from nodes partially replaced by metastatic tumour. In cancer of the breast, regional lymph nodes responded to PHA more vigorously than blood lymphocytes; both reacted more or less equally in patients with colonic cancers.

(4) Vánky and his colleagues have compared the reactivity of lymph node cells and blood lymphocytes against autologous tumour in an *in vitro* procedure akin to a mixed lymphocyte test (Stjernswärd and Vánky, 1972; Vánky *et al.*, 1973). In a group of patients with large sarcomas, local lymph node cells were found to be unreactive against the autologous tumour though some reactions were obtained with autologous blood lymphocytes. The basis for this discordant response is not clear. More experience with parallel investigations of blood lymphocytes and regional lymph node cells is clearly needed, particularly with tumours which (unlike sarcomas) regularly metastasise to local nodes.

(5) Lymphocyte migration inhibition assays have been studied by Ellis *et al.* (1975), using cells from axillary lymph nodes and blood lymphocytes in patients with breast cancer. A significant response was found with 17/24 regional lymph nodes as compared with 7/24 peripheral blood samples, suggesting a more vigorously reacting cell population in the draining nodes.

(6) Several authors have reported qualitative *in vitro* studies of interactions between tumour cells, maintained in short-term culture, and autologous lymph node cells (Richters and Sherwin, 1971; Sherwin and Richters, 1972; Deodhar *et al.*, 1972). With breast cancers, the observed patterns included clustering of lymphocytes round tumour cells, emperipolesis and—in the investigation of Deodhar and his colleagues—transformation of lymphocytes and actual destruction of tumour cells. Sherwin and Richters were unable to detect any differences when the lymphocytes were obtained from uninvolved or from partially involved nodes; Deodhar *et al.* found less interaction with lymphocytes from nodes containing secondary tumour. Such investigations are difficult to control and more quantitative techniques are preferable.

Morphological and functional studies in lymph nodes draining tumours in experimental animals have been widely reported. Most of the tumours have, however, been transplanted lesions, few of which metastasise.

Working with a syngeneic squamous cell carcinoma in rats, Flannery *et al.* (1973) showed that antitumour activity, measured by *in vitro* cytotoxicity, reached a peak in the draining nodes about two weeks after tumour transplantation. Acitivity then declined in the local nodes but cytotoxic cells became demonstrable in more distal sites, indicating a systemization of the immune response. The anergic phase in the regional nodes coincided with the development of distant metastases. These results are summarized in Fig. 2.

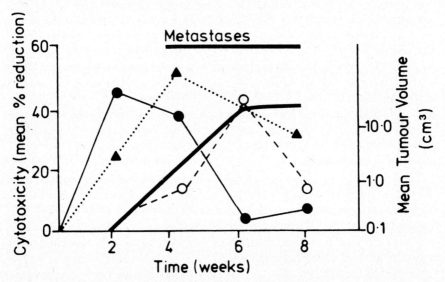

FIG. 2. Development of cytotoxic lymphocytes in a rat grafted with a syngeneic squamous carcinoma. Cytotoxic activity plotted for cells from the regional lymph node (●———●), a distant node (O – – – O), and from blood (▲ . . . . ▲). The heavy continuous line (———) represents the volume of the tumour graft. Redrawn from data from Flannery *et al.* (1973)

Other experimental tumour models have given a less clear-cut picture. It is uncertain, for example, whether the late anergic phase in the regional nodes is specific (compare Rowland *et al.*, 1971; Flannery *et al.*, 1973). In some systems there appears to be little or no anergy, cells in the draining nodes retaining their antitumour activity until the animals are virtually moribund (Fisher *et al.*, 1974). Despite the sustained reactivity of cells in the draining nodes, the tumour grafts grew progressively in these experiments; but the absence of lymph node metastases suggests that local cytotoxic cells may have destroyed individual tumour cells which reached the node. Thirdly, antitumour activity in *distant* lymphoid structures or in blood lymphocytes varies in strength and time course (cf. Goldfarb and Hardy, 1975). The effects of experimental tumours on the lymphoid system are obviously variable and highly complex, and the inter-related factors of tumour size, the rate of tumour growth and the duration of tumour appear crucial (Burk et al., 1975).

Changes in T and B cell populations in nodes draining experimental tumours are not well documented. Weston and her colleagues (1972, 1974) have studied the responses evoked by the EL4 lymphoma, growing as solid allografts in chimaeric CBA mice and in T cell deprived animals. Reconstituted mice mount a brisk paracortical reaction in the regional lymph nodes though the response tends to be abnormal in both intensity and time course (see Weston et al., 1972 for details). The peak of paracortical T cell activity coincided with the accumulation of lymphoid cells within the tumour grafts and a temporary slowing of growth of the transplants; no metastases developed. When similar experiments were made with T cell *deficient* mice, unable to mount a paracortical response, the local EL4 grafts grew progressively, no local infiltrates developed and metastases

TABLE 1

Metastases from EL4 lymphoma[a] in normal and T cell deficient (deprived) CBA mice

	Normal	T cell deficient
Time of death	—	20–26 days
	(killed at 26 days)	
Autopsies	10	22
Metastases	0/10	11/22
kidneys	0	8
liver	0	6
spleen	0	2
adrenals	0	2
duodenum	0	1
anterior mediastinum	0	1
[Regional lymph nodes[b]	0	0]
[Lungs[b]	0	0]

[a] EL4 lymphoma (2×10^6 cells) transplanted intradermally into flank.
[b] Note absence of metastases in regional lymph nodes and lungs in T cell deficient mice. (Data from Weston et al., 1974).

appeared in about 50% of mice (*see* Table 1). As the tumour allografts grew more quickly in T cell deficient animals, further investigations were made in which EL4 cells were injected intravenously into three groups of CBA mice: normal, T cell-deficient and T cell reconstituted. Differences in the amount and distribution of tumour deposits were seen in T cell deficient mice as compared with the normal or T cell-reconstituted groups—Table 2. The difference in anatomical distribution is particularly interesting; the possible contribution made by immune factors in the complex matter of localization of metastatic tumour was discussed earlier in Chapter I.

These observations suggest that T cells are in some way implicated in the control of metastatic growth, a view that is supported by other lines of evidence. Studies with syngeneic 3,4-benzpyrene-induced

TABLE 2

Deposits from EL4 cells (2×10^6) injected intravenously into normal, T cell deficient (deprived) and T cell reconstituted CBA mice

	Normal	T cell deficient	T cell reconstituted
Time of death (days)	28–106[a]	14–16	28–82 (mean 48)
Autopsies	12	15	10
Tumour deposits	9/12[b]	15/15[c]	6/10[b]
liver	1	15	0
kidneys	0	15	1
adrenals	0	9	0
spleen	0	6	0
lymph nodes	0	0	0
duodenum	0	2	0
lungs	1	6	1
Caudal muscles	1	0	0
Posterior abdominal wall	5	0	1
Diaphragm	1	0	0
Posterior thoracic wall	1	0	2
Interscapular region	1	0	2
Orbit	0	0	1

[a] Three normal mice, free of tumour, were killed at 206 days.
[b] Normal and T cell reconstituted mice: tumour deposits few, small and mainly localized in *soft tissues*. Typically circumscribed lesions surrounded by dense infiltrates of host cells.
[c] T cell deficient mice: tumour cell deposits numerous, large and localized exclusively to *viscera*. Typically diffuse lesions with little or no associated infiltrate of host cells. (Data from Weston *et al.*, 1974).

fibrosarcomas in rats have shown that metastasis is enhanced in animals whose T cell levels have been depleted by chronic thoracic duct drainage or by thymectomy and whole body irradiation (Eccles and Alexander, 1974, 1975). Treatment with antithymocyte serum enhances the incidence of metastasis from a variety of autochthonous and allogeneic tumours in rats, mice and hamsters—Fig. 3 (*see also* Deodhar and Crile, 1969; Fisher *et al.*, 1969; Gershon and Carter, 1970); so, too, does neonatal thymectomy or adult thymectomy plus irradiation in mice (Carnaud *et al.*, 1974) and thymectomy and

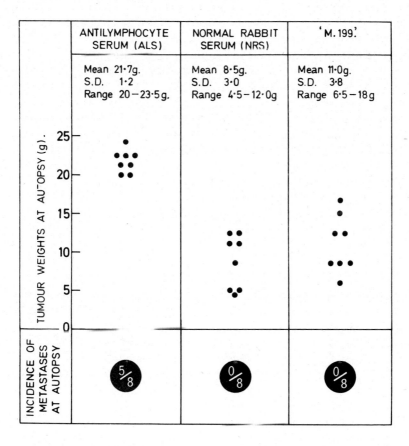

FIG. 3. Tumour weights and incidence of metastases from NML, grafted subcutaneously in hamsters treated with antilymphocyte serum (ALS), normal rabbit serum (NRS) or culture medium ('M 199'). The tumour grafts removed from ALS-treated animals are larger and show less variation in weight than in the control groups, suggesting that tumour growth is more uniform when the immune response is suppressed. Metastases from NML were found in axillary, mediastinal and para-aortic lymph nodes and in the periscapular brown fat

splenectomy in rats (Kim, 1970. The observations of Carnaud *et al.*
are interesting as these workers showed that immunological restoration of "depleted" mice, either by injecting lymphoid cells or by
thymus grafting, significantly reduced the number of metastases as
compared with the number in otherwise similar "depleted" mice.
Primary tumours may themselves exert an immunosuppressive
effect, possibly with selective inhibition of T cell activity (Haba *et al.*,
1976).

Certain cautionary points must, however, be noted. Some
immunosuppressive measures such as whole body irradiation and
corticosteroid treatment have widespread and often poorly-localized
effects both within the immune system and outside it. Immunosuppression, in some experimental models, has failed to enhance
metastatic growth or has given rise to conflicting results (Boeryd and
Suurküla, 1973; Suurküla and Boeryd, 1974). Human tumours,
growing as xenografts in (congenitally) T cell deficient nude mice,
very rarely metastasise (Giovanella *et al.*, 1973). The potentiating
effects of artificial T cell deprivation on metastasis are most clearly
seen with allogeneic tumours (Woodruff *et al.*, 1973). Lastly, the
mode of action of T cells in allogeneic or syngeneic tumour systems is
ill understood, and the T cell deficient state involves not only a
quantitative deficit of cytotoxic T cells but also a disturbance in T
and B cell co-operation and a lack of T cell-associated products
(lymphokines).

A. *Excision of Regional Lymph Nodes*

The preceding sections have indicated that at least some tumours
evoke morphologic responses in the local nodes at certain stages of
their development, and that such responses may (at least temporarily) be inimical to the tumour's progressive growth. These
observations impinge on the matter of practical management of
uninvolved regional lymph nodes in cancer patients, and constitute a
topic which remains one of the major controversies in clinical and
experimental oncology.

The controversy has stemmed largely from the studies of Crile
(1965, 1968, 1969, 1975). Briefly summarizing the experimental work
in mice, Crile has reported that early excision of small transplanted
tumours (allogeneic and syngeneic) together with the regional lymph
nodes has deleterious effects—a high incidence of metastases to other
nodes or to the lungs (or both), and increased susceptibility to
rechallenge with the same tumour.

Investigations by Fisher and Fisher (1971, 1972; also Fisher *et al.*, 1974) have provided evidence that the regional nodes play a major role in the initiation and maintenance of immunity to a syngeneic mammary tumour in C3H mice—but not, significantly, in a strongly immunogenic methylcholanthrene-induced fibrosarcoma in the same strain. On the other hand, several workers have failed to confirm Crile's findings (Bard *et al.*, 1969; Bard and Pilch, 1969; Hammond and Rolley, 1970; McCredie *et al.*, 1973). Many of these studies have the advantage of the use of recently induced syngeneic tumours, particularly mammary adenocarcinomas; but the tumours have often been larger and excised later than in Crile's experiments. Crile's own observations certainly tally with the classical study of Mitchison (1954) in which he demonstrated that, for about 5 to 15 days after tumour transplantation, immune reactivity remained largely localized to the draining nodes as shown by successful adoptive transfer of immunity with lymph node cells. Later on, Mitchison found that adoptive transfer of immunity from the local node was increasingly ineffective.

It is questionable whether Crile's results of early excision have any clinical counterpart. Given that most human tumours probably develop rather slowly, it is difficult to imagine that an immune response, even though initiated in the regional nodes, has not systematized throughout the immune system by the time that most patients first present clinically. The diversity of tumours (and their regional lymph nodes) should also be stressed. The merits of prophylactic dissection of axillary lymph nodes draining a carcinoma of the breast are disputed, but the case for irradiating pelvic and abdominal nodes draining a testicular seminoma is now widely accepted.

IV. Studies on Metastasising and Non-metastasising Lymphomas (ML and NML) in Hamsters

The lymphoreticular responses to metastasising tumours have been investigated with a pair of hamster lymphomas in a series of papers from Yale and London dating back to 1966 (Carter and Gershon, 1966, 1967; Gershon and Carter, 1967, 1970; Carter *et al.*, 1968; Gershon *et al.*, 1967a, b, 1968; Nomoto *et al.*, 1970; Birbeck and Carter, 1972; Machinami *et al.*, 1975).

The salient features of the metastasising and non-metastasising lymphomas are summarized in Table 3.

TABLE 3

Some general characteristics of a non-metastasising lymphoma (NML) and a metastasising lymphoma (ML) in hamsters

	NML	ML
Source	"Spontaneous"	"Spontaneous"
Histology[a]	Diffuse lymphoblastic lymphoma	Diffuse lymphoblastic lymphoma
Transplantation as cell suspensions or solid fragments	Readily transplanted	Readily transplanted
Growth at site of transplantation	Rapid	Rapid
Viable tumour cells in blood[b]	+	+
Viable tumour cells in regional lymph nodes[c]	+	+
Metastases[d]	–	+
Effect of rechallenge with second graft of the same tumour[e]	New graft rejected	New graft accepted

[a] ML and NML cells are virtually indistinguishable in the light microscope but NML is characteristically infiltrated with macrophages while ML is not (*see* text). Both tumours are also closely similar in the electron microscope except that some ML cells contain small stacks of rough endoplasmic reticulum. ML cells contain abundant surface immunoglobulin demonstrable by immunofluorescence and, in the electron microscope, by immuno-peroxidase techniques; NML cells lack surface immunoglobulins.

[b,c] Presence of viable tumour cells assessed crudely by transplanting whole blood (b) or cell suspensions of regional lymph nodes (c) into the subcutaneous tissues of normal hamsters. Lymphomas develop at the site of inoculation usually within 20 days.

[d] *NML*: Although individual viable cells are present for some time in the draining lymph nodes, foci of metastatic tumour do not develop.
   ML: Microscopic and macroscopic deposits of confluent tumour develop consistently in the draining nodes and also in mediastinal nodes, thymus and liver; other sites are less often affected such as the contralateral axillary nodes, inguinal nodes, mesenteric nodes and kidneys.

[e] NML elicits a state of concomitant immunity and no metastases develop unless immunity is broken by irradiation or treatment with ATS. No concomitant immunity is seen with ML.

The two tumours share an almost identical morphology in both the light and electron microscope and are most easily distinguished not by the appearances of the neoplastic cells but by the infiltrate of activated macrophages which is found in NML (Gershon *et al.*, 1967a; Birbeck and Carter, 1972).

Subcutaneous grafts of the two tumours evoke strikingly different morphological reactions in the draining lymph nodes which are summarized in Table 4. Detailed morphological descriptions are given in Carter and Gershon (1966, 1967), Gershon and Carter (1967), Gershon *et al*. (1967a) and Carter *et al*. (1968). In brief, the response to NML in the *regional nodes* is dominated by paracortical hyperplasia and sinus histiocytosis, followed by follicular activation. The sinus histiocytes are markedly phagocytic and appear to ingest tumour cells (*see* Fig. 5B in *Chapter I*). No metastatic deposits are established. By contrast, ML evokes little change in the paracortex and sinuses of the regional nodes, and the principal feature is

TABLE 4

Morphological changes in regional lymph nodes evoked by grafts of NML and ML

	NML	ML
	Draining nodes	
Tumour cells	Appear early; localized to sinuses; no metastatic deposits formed	Appear late; spread throughout sinuses and pulp to form confluent deposits
Sinus system	Prominent sinus histiocytosis; + +phago- cytosis of erythrocytes and tumour cells[a]	Negligible sinus histiocytosis. Little or no phagocytic activity
T cell zone: paracortex	Hyperplasia of pyroninophilic blast cells	Little response
B cell zones: follicles	Enlarged and active during later stages	Generally inactive
medullary cords	Moderately enlarged. Pleomorphic cell constituents	Massive plasmacytosis[b]

[a] Macrophages appear to assist immune lymphoid cells in the destruction of NML; despite their prominence they are not the primary effector cell.
[b] Plasma cells in the medullary cords contain abundant stainable immunoglobulin. Similar material is also present on the surface of ML, but not NML, cells (cf. Table 3).

proliferation of immunoglobulin-containing plasma cells in the medullary cords which persist until the nodes are replaced by confluent metastatic deposits. Neither tumour evokes reactive changes in the *contralateral nodes*, and the *spleen* shows essentially non-specific morphological responses in the red and white pulp, more marked in animals grafted with NML. If the regional lymph nodes are excised before either tumour is grafted, the appropriate morphological changes develop in the next nodes in the drainage system with no alteration in biological behaviour.

For ML, the histological changes appear to be those of a B cell response which is dominated by plasma cell proliferation and immunoglobulin production. Stainable immunoglobulin is also present on the surface of ML cells (though some of this immuno-globulin may perhaps be synthesized *locally* by the tumour as an intrinsic, self-generating mechanism to potentiate metastatic growth). Experiments in which the effects of various combinations of ML and NML, given together or sequentially, indicate that the absence of sinus histiocytosis in ML-bearing hamsters is not due to any suppression of histiocytes by the tumour (Gershon and Carter, 1967; Carter and Gershon, 1967).

For NML, the histological response appears to show a mixed T and B cell pattern, the former predominating. In contrast to the findings with ML, nodes draining NML remain morphologically normal until tumour cells begin to appear in the peripheral sinuses. There is then a generalized reaction first involving paracortical cells and sinus histiocytes. Follicles in the B cell zone are activated later but there is little response in the medullary cords (cf. ML). Cellular reactions in the paracortex and sinuses appear to be linked in time, but the mechanisms which underlie sinus histiocytosis are unknown. The sinus histiocytosis found in nodes draining NML differs in certain respects from the sinus histiocytosis described in nodes draining human tumours such as breast, stomach and colon. In the hamsters, sinus histiocytosis is only apparent *after* tumour cells begin to accumulate in the sinuses; secondly, phagocytosis of tumour cells has not been described in human lymph nodes. Although phagocytosis is a striking feature in the response elicited by NML, it is important to note that macrophages apparently do not assist immune lymphoid cells in killing NML cells (Nomoto *et al.*, 1970).

Functional aspects of the immune response evoked by NML have been studied, and it has been shown that the tumour induces a state of *concomitant immunity* (Gershon *et al.*, 1967b). As an NML allograft grows, the animal develops a high degree of tumour immunity which

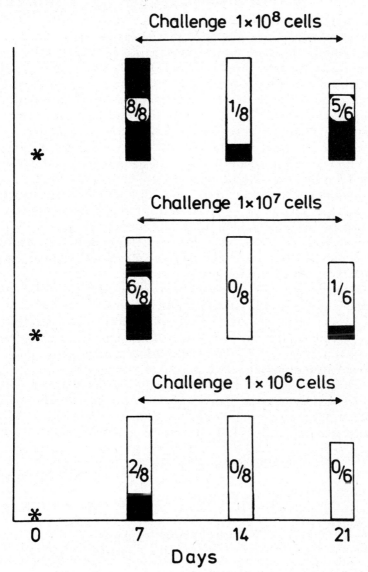

FIG. 4. Development and strength of concomitant immunity in hamsters bearing grafts of NML. All animals received an immunizing graft of 1×10^7 NML cells in the subcutaneous tissues of the flank on day 0 (marked ∗). A challenge of 1×10^6 or 1×10^7 or 1×10^8 NML cells was given subcutaneously into the opposite flank on day 7 or day 14 or day 21.

is specific and cell-mediated (see Fig. 4). Paradoxically, this developing immunity co-exists with the progressively growing tumour graft which provoked it; but if the animal is re-challenged with the same tumour, the new graft will be promptly rejected, a process in which macrophages play a major part. There is no demonstrable cross-immunity between NML and ML, and no concomitant immunity has been described with ML.

The proposal that concomitant immunity may play a role in preventing the establishment of metastases from NML is underlined by the finding that NML *will* metastasise in hamsters where concomitant immunity is abrogated by whole body irradiation or, more specifically by antithymocyte serum—*see* Fig. 3. More problematically, NML may also metastasise if the immunizing tumour graft is excised within certain time-limits (Gershon *et al.*, 1968).

Concomitant immunity has been described experimentally in rats, mice and hamsters in relation to spontaneous tumours and to tumours induced with chemicals and viruses (Nelson, 1974). T cells are probably involved, and the process appears to provide a mechanism which prevents or impedes the establishment and growth of metastases from certain kinds of tumour.

Two cautionary points should be noted in relation to the findings in hamsters. Both ML and NML are allografts—though it will be recalled that hamsters are anomalous in terms of tissue transplantation because they have very few detectable histo-compatibility genes (Billingham *et al.*, 1960). Secondly, the characterization of T and B cell responses has been based largely on indirect morphological grounds and responses in carefully characterized T cell deficient animals need to be investigated: it has already been emphasized that the macrophage response, though prominent, is essentially secondary to a direct attack on NML by lymphoid cells (Nomoto *et al.*, 1970).

References

Alderson, M. R., Hamlin, I. and Staunton, M. D. (1971. *Brit. J. Cancer*, **25**, 646–656.

Alexander, P. (1976). *In* "Fundamental Aspects of Metastasis" (L. Weiss, ed.), pp. 227–239. North-Holland Publishing Company, Amsterdam-Oxford.

Anastassiades, O. T. and Pryce, D. M. (1966). *Brit. J. Cancer*, **20**, 239–249.

Bard, D. S. and Pilch, Y. H. (1969). *Cancer Res.* **29**, 1125–1131.

Bard, D. S., Hammond, W. G. and Pilch, H. (1969). *Cancer Res.* **29**, 1379–1384.

Bennett, S. H., Futrell, J. W., Roth, J. A., Hoye, R. C. and Ketcham, A. S. (1971). *Cancer, Philad.* **28**, 1255–1265.

Berlinger, N. T., Tsakraklides, V., Pollak, K., Adams, G.L., Yang, M. and Good, R. A. (1976). *Laryngoscope (St. Louis)*, **87**, 792–803.

Billingham, R. E., Sawchuck, G. H. and Silvers, W. K. (1960). *Proc. Nat. Acad. Sci. (Wash.)*, **46**, 1079–1090.

Birbeck, M. S. C. and Carter, R. L. (1972). *Int. J. Cancer*, 9, 249–257.

Black, M. M., Freeman, C., Mork, T., Harvei, S. and Cutler, S. J. (1971). *Cancer, Philad.* 27, 703–711.

Black, M. M., Kerpe, S. and Speer, F. D. (1953). *Amer. J. Path.* 29, 505–521.

Black, M. M., Opler, S. R. and Speer, F. D. (1954). *Surg. Gynec. Obstet.* 98, 725–734.

Black, M. M., Opler, S. R. and Speer, F. D. (1955). *Surg. Gynec. Obstet.* 100, 543–551.

Boeryd, B. and Suurküla, M. (1973). *Int. J. Cancer*, 12, 722–727.

Burk, M. W., Yu. S., Ristow, S. S. and McKhann, C. F. (1975). *Int. J. Cancer*, 15, 99–108.

Burtin, P., Loisillier, F., Buffe, D., Guillerm, M. and Gluckman, E. (1969). *Cancer, Philad.* 23, 80–87.

Carnaud, C., Hoch, B. and Trainin, N. (1974). *J. Natl. Cancer Inst.* 52, 395–399.

Carr, I. and Underwood, J. C. E. (1974). *Int. Rev. Cytol.* 37, 329–347.

Carter, R. L. and Gershon, R. K. (1966). *Amer. J. Path.* 49, 637–655.

Carter, R. L. and Gershon, R. K. (1967). *Amer. J. Path.* 50, 203–217.

Carter, R. L., Gershon, R. K. and Kondo, K. (1968). *Transplantation*, 6, 313–321.

Carter, R. L. (1975a). Metastasis. *In* "Biology of Cancer" (E. J. Ambrose and F. J. C. Roe, eds), pp. 74–95. 2nd edn. Ellis Horwood, Chichester.

Carter, R. L. (1975b). *In* "Host Defence in Breast Cancer" (B. Stoll, ed.), pp. 6–35. William Heinemann, Medical Books Ltd., London.

Crile, G., Jr. (1965). *Surg. Gynec. Obstet.* 120, 975–982.

Crile, G., Jr. (1968). *Surg. Gynec. Obstet.* 126, 1270–1272.

Crile, G., Jr. (1969). *Cancer, Philad.* 24, 1283–1285.

Crile, G., Jr. (1975). *In* "Host Defences in Breast Cancer", Vol. 1 (B. Stoll, ed.), pp. 121–129. William Heinemann Medical Books, London.

Deodhar, S. D. and Crile, G., Jr. (1969). *Cancer Res.* 29, 776–779.

Deodhar, S. D., Crile, G., Jr. and Esselstyn, C. B., Jr. (1972). *Cancer, Philad.* 29, 1321–1325.

Eccles, S. A. and Alexander, P. (1974). *Nature, Lond.* 250, 667–669.

Eccles, S. A. and Alexander, P. (1975). *Nature, Lond.* 257, 52–53.

Ellis, R. J., Wernick, G., Zobriskie, J. B. and Goldman, L. I. (1975). *Cancer, Philad.* 35, 655–659.

Fisher, B. and Fisher, E. R. (1971). *Cancer, Philad.* 27, 1001–1004.

Fisher, B. and Fisher, E. R. (1972). *Cancer, Philad.* 29, 1496–1501.

Fisher, B., Soliman, O. and Fisher, E. R. (1969). *Proc. Soc. exp. Biol. Med.* 131, 16–18.

Fisher, B., Saffer, E. A. and Fisher, E. R. (1972). *Cancer, Philad.* 30, 1202–1215.

Fisher, B., Saffer, E. A. and Fisher, E. R. (1974). *Cancer, Philad.* 33, 631–636.

Flannery, G. R., Chalmers, R. J., Rolland, J. M. and Nairn, R. C. (1973). *Brit. J. Cancer*, 28, 118–122.

Gershon, R. K. and Carter, R. L. (1967). *Amer. J. Path.* 50, 137–157.

Gershon, R. K. and Carter, R. L. (1970). *Nature, Lond.* 226, 368–370.

Gershon, R. K., Carter, R. L. and Lane, N. J. (1967a). *Amer. J. Path.* 51, 1111–1133.

Gershon, R. K., Carter, R. L. and Kondo, K. (1967b). *Nature, Lond.* 213, 674–676.

Gershon, R. K., Carter, R. L. and Kondo, K. (1968). *Science*, 159, 646–648.

Giovanella, B. C., Yim, S. O., Morgan, A. C., Stehlin, J. S. and Williams, L. J., Jr. (1973). *J. Natl. Cancer Inst.* 50, 1051–1053.

Goldfarb, P. M. and Hardy, M. A. (1975). *Cancer, Philad.* 35, 778–783.

Haba, S., Hamaoka, T., Takatsa, K. and Kitagawa, M. (1976). *Int. J. Cancer*, **18**, 93–104.

Hamlin, I. M. E. (1968). *Brit. J. Cancer*, **22**, 383–401.

Hammond, W. G. and Rolley, R. T. (1970). *Cancer, Philad.* **25**, 368–372.

Kerbel, R. S. and Davies, A. J. S. (1974). *Cell*, **3**, 105–112.

Kerbel, R. S., Pross, H. F. and Elliott, E. V. (1975). *Int. J. Cancer*, **15**, 918–930.

Kim, U. (1970). *Science*, **167**, 72–74.

Machinami, R., Carter, R. L. and Birbeck, M. S. C. (1975). *Europ. J. Cancer*, **11**, 87–90.

McCredie, J. A., Inch, W. R. and Cowie, H. C. (1973). *Cancer, Philad.* **31**, 983–987.

Mitchison, N. A. (1954). *Proc. R. Soc. Ser. B.* **142**, 72–87.

Nelson, D. S. (1974). *Transplant. Rev.* **19**, 226–254.

Nomoto, K., Gershon, R. K. and Waksman, B. H. (1970). *J. Natl. Cancer Inst.* **44**, 739–747.

Patt, D. J., Brynes, R. K., Vardiman, J. W. and Coppleston, L. W. (1975). *Cancer, Philad.* **35**, 1388–1397.

Richters, A. and Sherwin, R. P. (1971). *Cancer, Philad.* **27**, 274–277.

Roubin, R., Cesarini, J-P., Fridman, W. H., Pavie-Fischer, J. and Peter, H. H. (1975). *Int. J. Cancer*, **16**, 61–73.

Rowland, G. F., Edwards, A. J., Hurd, C. M. and Sumner, M. R. (1971). *J. Natl. Cancer Inst.* **47**, 321–327.

Sherwin, R. P. and Richters, A. (1972). *J. Natl. Cancer Inst.* **48**, 1111–1115.

Snyderman, R., Pike, M. C., Blaylock, B. L. and Weinstein, P. (1976). *J. Immunol.* **116**, 585–589.

Stjernswärd, J. and Vánky, F. (1972). *Nat. Cancer Inst. Monogr.* **35**, 237–242.

Suurküla, M. and Boeryd, B. (1974). *Int. J. Cancer*, **14**, 633–641.

Tsakraklides, V., Tsakraklides, E. and Good, R. A. (1975a). *Amer. J. Path.* **78**, 7–22.

Tsakraklides, E., Tsakraklides, V., Ashikari, H., Rosen, P. P., Segal, F. P., Robbins, G. F. and Good, R. A. (1975c). *J. Natl. Cancer Inst.* **54**, 549–556.

Tsakraklides, V., Anastassiades, D. T. and Kersey, J. H. (1973). *Cancer, Philad.* **31**, 860–869.

Tsakraklides, V., Olson, P., Kersey, J. H. and Good, R. A. (1974). *Cancer, Philad.* **34**, 1259–1267.

Tsakraklides, V., Wanebo, H. J., Sternberg, S. S., Stearns, M. and Good, R. A. (1975b). *Amer. J. Surg.* **129**, 174–180.

Turner, D. R. and Berry, C. L. (1972). *J. clin. Path.* **25**, 1053–1055.

Underwood, J. C. E. and Carr, I. (1972). *Virchow's Arch. path. Anat. Abt. B.* **12**, 39.

Underwood, J. C. E. (1974). *Brit. J. Cancer*, **30**, 538–548.

Vánky, F., Stjernswärd, J., Nilsonne, U. and Sundblad, R. (1973). *J. Natl. Cancer Inst.* **51**, 17–24.

Weston, B. J., Cheers, C., Carter, R. L., Leuchars, E., Wallis, V. J. and Davies, A. J. S. (1972). *Int. J. Cancer*, **9**, 66–75.

Weston, B. J., Carter, R. L., Easty, G. C., Connell, D. I. and Davies, A. J. S. (1974). *Int. J. Cancer*, **14**, 176–185.

Wood, G. W. and Gillespie, G. Y. (1975). *Int. J. Cancer*, **16**, 1022–1029.

Woodruff, M., Dunbar, N. and Ghaffar, A. (1973). *Proc. R. Soc. Ser. B.* **184**, 97–102.

Chapter III

Radiotherapy and Metastases

C. F. VON ESSEN* AND J. STJERNSWÄRD†

* *Swiss Institute of Nuclear Research, 5234 Villigen, Switzerland*
† *Ludwig Institute for Cancer Research (Lausanne Branch)*
and Dept. of Radiotherapy, Cantonal University Hospital
Lausanne, Switzerland

I. Radiotherapy and Metastasis

Radiation therapy continues to progress as an effective curative and palliative treatment of many forms of cancer. From 40 to 50% of all patients with cancer receive radiation therapy at some time in the course of the disease (Stein, 1973). Rates of long-term remission, considered an index of curability, approach 100% in several sites, particularly at early stages. Many reviews of the current status of radiation therapy in cancer treatment are available for reference (Fletcher, 1973). This chapter will deal only with the role of ionizing radiation in metastatic cancer.

Radiation therapy, similarly to surgery, is considered a local treatment for regionally limited cancer. Systemic treatment by whole body irradiation, however, may also have some value in the treatment of disseminated disease. The relationship between the radiation dose required to ablate a cancerous deposit and the dose which will result in severe damage to normal tissues or even death of the patient is tumour volume dependent and inversely tissue volume dependent respectively (von Essen, 1963). As the radiated tissue volume increases the normal tissues become more susceptible to damage because of reduction of cell viability below critical limits and interference with repopulation. Radiation of the total body is associated with the 50% human lethal single dose of the order of 600 rads, while the single dose required to sterilize even 90% of the cells in large tumour volume is of the order of many thousand rads. This negative therapeutic ratio can be modified somewhat by fractionation and protraction of the dose in order to exploit possible differences between normal and malignant cells, including repair of sub-lethal damage and reoxygenation (reviewed by Suit, 1973). Thus from a theoretical radiobiological basis there appears to be little role for systemic radiation therapy in the curative treatment of disseminated cancer, although some promising approaches are being made in the curative treatment of leukemias utilizing bone marrow transplantation after radiation (Thomas *et al.*, 1973) and using total body irradiation of lymphomas (Johnson, 1975; Loeffler and Puterbaugh, 1975), both of these tumour types being considered radiosensitive.

There are however, other roles of radiation therapy in the control of metastatic disease. One is the planned use of radiation in conjunction with surgery in order to improve the control rate of cancers that tend to extend microscopically beyond the scope of surgical excision. The other is the use of radiation in the treatment of specific sites at high risk for metastatic disease, generally leukemias existing in "sanctuaries" beyond the reach of bloodborn chemotherapeutic drugs. Finally, the *palliative* treatment of existing and symptomatic metastasis represents one of the most important contributions of radiation therapy to cancer management.

However, despite these potential and actual positive contributions, there have been numerous reports of a different nature: the effect of radiation therapy to enhance the incidence and growth of metastasis. These studies have been based on largely experimental animal tumour systems, but clinical data appear to indicate that some of these effects, at least, are of clinical significance (Stjernswärd, 1974).

We will analyse these data seeking to answer the question whether implantation and growth of metastasis may be stimulated by irradiation of the primary tumour site as well as of distant tissues under certain circumstances.

Another aspect to be reviewed is the significance of the data that radiotherapy, even when given as a localized form of therapy, has a systemic effect on the host, e.g. in producing a long lasting lymphopenia. This may be of importance in a situation where circulating cancer cells are already established and undetectable micro-metastases are present.

An analysis of available experimental data as well as results from existing controlled clinical trials will be given in order to help to define the role of radiotherapy in the secondary spread of cancer as outlined above. These aspects include the rationale for pre-operative radiotherapy and post-operative radiotherapy, prophylactic radiotherapy of the lung in certain neoplastic states, and the radiation of the central nervous system in leukemia.

The current role of radiation therapy in the management of disseminated cancer will be discussed, as well as a critical review and analysis of the evidence that radiation therapy may play a beneficial or a harmful role under certain conditions in the dissemination of cancer.

II. Beneficial Effects of Irradiation

The therapeutic ratio of radiotherapy is constantly being improved and the present pathways for doing this will be briefly outlined. Some of these developments affect not only the primary but also the secondary spread of cancer. They consist of:

1. Increasing the normal tissue tolerence to irradiation.
2. Increasing tumour response to irradiation by
   (a) radio sensitizers,
   (b) improved radiation by using particles such as neutrons, pi-mesons and heavy ions,
   (c) hyperthermia,
   (d) hyperbaric oxygen,
   (e) optimal biological fractionation schedules.
3. Combination therapy between surgery and radiotherapy, radiotherapy and chemotherapy, radiotherapy and immuno-therapy.
4. Elective treatment of sub-clinical disease.
5. Sanctuary irradiation.

6. Fractionated whole body or sub-total body irradiation.

The important curative role of radiotherapy in the management of well localized primary tumours will not be analysed as we are limiting ourselves to secondary spread.

Radiotherapy has a clear role in the management of secondary spread already established. It is used for elective treatment of sub-clinical disease in defined high risk groups, for palliation of clinical metastasis, to reach secondary spread in anatomically, pharmacologically, or immunologically privilege sanctuaries, as an effective cytotoxic agent in total body irradiation, and lately in combination therapy with chemotherapy.

Radiotherapy thus has a demonstrated positive role in the control of secondary spread despite being a localized form of therapy and despite the fact that distant metastases represent the major cause of failure in cancer therapy, except for tumours of the central nervous system and head and neck.

Radiation therapy is unlikely to solve the problem of failure of distant metastases, since doses tolerated by the whole body are insufficient in controlling even early sub-clinical metastatic disease of solid tumour. The combination of local and systemic therapy, e.g. irradiation/surgery with chemotherapy, hormonetherapy and/or immunotherapy is the logical way of improving survival. Chemotherapy together with irradiation for controlling known sub-clinical disease has led to some major therapeutical advancements in Wilm's tumour, embryonal rhabdomyosarcoma, Ewing's tumour, osteogenic sarcomas medulloblastoma and breast cancer. (Evans, 1975; Ghavimi et al., 1975; Rosen et al., 1974; Bloom et al., 1969; Nissen-Meyer, 1975). Combinations of radiation-chemotherapy offers a realistic pathway for not only preventing and curing metastasis but also enhancing the control of local-regional disease.

Sanctuary irradiation, e.g. in leukemias, has contributed to one of the recent major success and therapeutic improvements in cancer therapy.

A. *Palliation of Clinical Metastasis*

Radiotherapy being a local therapy, as is surgery, is used for curative intent in well-defined local tumours with or without regional metastasis. Radiotherapy has also a primary role in the treatment of secondary spread, when there are single metastases, or for palliation of symptomatic metastases. There are hardly any contra-indications for irradiation of bone metastases. For pulmonary metastases, radiotherapy may sometimes be more hazardous and lead to an impairment of pulmonary function. Radiation of lymph node metastases, as for instance supra-clavicular nodes, may result in secondary complications, such as damage of neural plexus with paresthesia and pain, limb oedema, and impaired shoulder movements. Improvement in neurological status after palliative irradiation of brain metastases is well documented (Order et al., 1968). The clinical experience is that radiotherapy is effective in relieving many of the distressing symptoms of progressive cancer, especially pain. A challenging therapeutic search has indicated that "half body" irradiation offers effective palliation in patients with symptomatic distant metastases, after all conventional methods of therapy have been exhausted (Fitzpatrick and Rider, 1976).

The effects of radiotherapy on metastases have often been historically accepted as therapeutically effective. However, few attempts have been made to determine whether there is a cost–benefit ratio that is advantageous when compared to simple analgesics, for example (Hall, 1976). As pointed out, little is known of the natural history of many of the malignant diseases where radiotherapy is used as a palliative form of treatment, to be able to evaluate whether objective beneficial effects are achieved. The natural evolution of the disease may show that there is no difference between irradiation and a placebo effect. This was found, indeed, following irradiation of benign changes (Goldie et al., 1970). Actually, no careful study has been made of the palliative benefit obtained by radiation therapy in comparison with that obtained by alternative methods in a clinical trial.

B. *Post- and Pre-operative Irradiation*

The rationales for post-operative irradiation are:

1. To decrease recurrences when a high local failure rate after surgery alone is known.
2. To treat known residual tumour.
3. To eradicate tumour growth in adjacent area, e.g. lymph nodes.

The rationales for pre-operative irradiation are:

1. To increase the possibility of resectability.
2. To diminish the radicality of surgery, and thus improve quality of life.

3. To diminish tumour implantation in the surgical site.
4. To decrease dissemination of viable tumour cells at the time of surgery.

With combined therapy, surgery could sometimes be less radical. Both post- and pre-operative radiotherapy thus provide the advantage of conservation of organs, functions and cosmesis, improving the quality of life for the patients, e.g. as in many cases of head and neck tumours.

The doubtful logic for using post- or pre-operative irradiation in patients with a known high frequency of sub-clinical distant spread, or with localized easily resectable tumours as well as the possible biological harmful effects of localized "prophylactic" irradiation will be analysed later.

Localized secondary spread of tumour is clearly decreased by post- and pre-operative irradiation, but in evaluating published clinical trials it is important to separate the beneficial effects locally from the final outcome, which often may depend on distant spread.

In breast cancer an excellent control of local regional disease is achieved post-operatively by irradiation (Montague and Nelson, 1975) without, however, improving survival; perhaps to the contrary (Stjernswärd, 1974) and very often with an increased morbidity like increased arm oedema and decreased shoulder mobility (Ainsfield, 1976; de Schryver, 1975). Soft tissue sarcoma with high local recurrence rate is an obvious candidate for post-operative radiotherapy. Irradiation has been reported to control synovial sarcoma and is strongly advocated post-operatively (Suit *et al.*, 1973). Head and neck cancers are another tumour group where radiotherapy diminishes the frequency of local spread and improves the quality of life (e.g. Strong *et al.*, 1966).

A logical question to ask regarding the role of radiotherapy in the treatment of primary tumour and regional secondary spread would be—as it is being done by the National Wilms Tumor Study in the USA—whether post-operative radiotherapy is necessary for patients with well incapsulated localized lesions after what appeared to be their total removal? In such patients there exists no difference after 2 years survival whether radiotherapy is added or not post-operatively, and to date only one of 100 patients within the Group I Wilms tumour have abdominal recurrence, in patients randomized to chemotherapy ± radiotherapy (Evans, 1975).

A prospective controlled trial (Higgins and Dwight, 1972) has demonstrated an increase survival and a reduced percentage of positive lymph nodes in the resected specimens after pre-operative irradiation for recto-sigmoid cancers. In lung cancer pre-operative irradiation did not improve the survival of patients with operable lung cancer. There appeared to be a harmful effect influencing the longevity of the resected group after irradiation (Roswit et al., 1970). The role of pre-operative irradiation in renal carcinoma is being studied in the USA in a national study involving irradiation pre-operatively (4500 rad/4–5 weeks) followed by nephrectomy. This therapy is possible because of high diagnostic accuracy of selective arteriography and nephrotomography which also may be supplemented by fine needle biopsy. Pre-operative radiotherapy has been recommended to all patients with kidney cancer where there is no evidence of distant metastases (Riches, 1968). Preliminary data in a small group of patients indicates that those with poorly differentiated hypernephroma particularly may benefit by pre-operative radiotherapy (Almgard et al., 1970). Readers are referred to a recent review updating the results of pre-operative irradiation and surgery in clinical studies (Potter, 1975) and to an earlier review outlining the logic for pre-operative irradiation (Perez, 1970).

C. Elective Irradiation of Sub-clinical Disease: Prophylactic Irradiation of the Lungs

Almost all patients with secondary spread to the lungs die in spite of removal of the primary. There is a "tumour free" interval when the patient has no clinically detectable lung tumour metastases. In such a situation it would be logical to irradiate the lung if we knew that the tumour cells were already lodged there at the time of operation or just afterwards, especially as we know that a therapeutical relationship exists between the dose of ionizing irradiation to a total tumour cell population, and the surviving fraction of these cells. However, if the tumour cells are not lodged in the lung but circulating freely and later nidating in the lung there would be a theoretical risk, both from the animal experiments and human empirical findings (see below), that an increased incidence of tumour metastases in the irradiated lung may occur. From the experimental point of view, the logical trial to answer this question would be to irradiate only one of the lungs. However, from the ethical point of view this is not possible. A clinical trial is en route within the EORTC, giving adjuvant irradiation to the whole lung post-operatively, to children with Ewing sarcoma and osteo sarcoma. To date there is definitely no indication of increased metastasis after megovoltage irradiation of both lungs, with a dose of about 2000 rads during 12 days in 10 sessions (Tubiana, 1976).

The factors which determine the final localization of metastatic lesions are not fully known. In one of our own breast cancer cases, cells started to grow 16 years after removal of the primary tumour in the skin of the pubic abdominal part of a patient who was irradiated for a secondary gynecological tumour. This indicates that:

(a) trapping and/or local outgrowth of tumour cells may be facilitated by certain rare circumstances in irradiated tissues, and

(b) tumour cells may have been circulating the whole time in this patient and nidated only later in a suitable area (Stjernswärd and Douglas, 1976).

D. *Hyperbaric Oxygen Therapy and Distant Metastases*

Some of the early data using hyperbaric oxygen therapy for cervix carcinoma Stage III and IV indicated an increase of distant metastases in the treated group. A review of the patients dying in the first six months showed that 25% of the patients in the hyperbaric group were dead with distant metastases whereas only 5% of the controlled group died from distant metastases (Johnson, 1965). Oxygen may be important in itself to the growth of the tumour independent of radiotherapy. Consequently it may be possible that the increased oxygenization may help the growth of distant metastases that are not irradiated. This study was not a randomized one and used earlier treated patients as controls. Later controlled trials have found that the frequency of distant metastases are identical in the groups treated with or without hyperbaric oxygen (Halnan, 1975; Dische, 1976).

The concept of increased spread or growth of secondary cancer in connection with irradiation in hyperbaric oxygen is thus not substantiated by controlled trials.

E. *Sanctuary Irradiation*

1. *Cerebro-spinal irradiation for reaching metastases in privileged sites*

The impressive improvement in the prognosis of ALL has been the result of two major developments:

(1) The more efficient use of chemotherapeutic agents, particularly the use of combinations of agents (Henderson, 1973).

(2) The prevention with irradiation of central nervous system relapses (Hustu *et al.*, 1973; Simone *et al.*, 1975).

Again, the difference in the immunosuppressive effect of radio-therapy as compared to chemotherapy, the former being longlasting the other temporary, sometimes even with an "overshoot phenomena (n)" (Serrou *et al.*, 1975) may have direct clinical and practical importance. There are no clinical or statistical differences between cerebro-spinal irradiation as compared to cerebral irradiation plus methothrexate intrathecally with regard to the frequency of relapses. However, the side effects were significantly more frequent in patients receiving cranio-spinal irradiation. Episodes of severe lymphopenia occurred about twice as often, and chemotherapy had to be interrupted more often, and for longer periods (Simone *et al.*, 1975). A Medical Research Council study (1973) has shown together with a study of the immunosuppressive consequences of radiotherapy and chemotherapy in patients with ALL (Campbell *et al.*, 1973) that lymphopenia was much more marked in those patients who had previously received irradiation. Patients that died of infection during remission were all in the irradiated group, while none of those treated with chemotherapy alone died in remission. Depending on whether a neutropenia or a lymphopenia occurred the death in remission could be attributed to viral or bacterial infections (Medical Research Council, 1975; Campbell *et al.*, 1973; MacLennan *et al.*, 1976 in press).

F. *Total or Sub-total Body Irradiation*

Total body irradiation is an effective cytotoxic agent. It will reach tumour cells in sanctuaries, it does not require the circulatory system to reach the tumour cells, and it is not influenced by the blood/brain barrier or by cell membrane permeability. It has been used with success in patients with widespread metastatic disease, specially chronic lymphatic leukemias (Johnson, 1976; del Regato, 1974), non-Hodgkins' lymphoma (Johnson, 1975). Sub-total irradiation may be beneficial with palliative results not only in lymphomas (Johnson, 1975) but also in metastatic solid tumours, such as breast and prostatic cancer (Loeffler and Puterbaugh, 1975; Fitzpatrick and Rider, 1976). Irradiation has the advantage of also killing cells in the Go phase. Total body irradiation, using a half-body technique with doses of 500 rad or more to half of the body, repeated to the other half a little later, offers a fascinating pathway to explore in the future as adjuvant treatment for occult disease in patients with a poor prognosis. Radiotherapy may here move forward and expand to be a systemic therapy leaving its present limitations of being only a localized treatment modality.

G. *Improvement of Local Therapeutic Ratio*

The improvement of the therapeutic ratio of radiotherapy by radio-sensitizers, chemical agents which have capacity to increase the lethal properties of ionizing radiation when administered in conjunction with irradiation, or by increased oxygenization, or by heavy particle radiation therapy using neutrons and pi-mesons—hopefully will increase the therapeutic ratio of radiotherapy in localized disease. Unfortunately, however, the majority of tumours at the present stage of diagnosis are already disseminated. Therefore, even if the above improvements will increase the therapeutic ratio, their overall effect on the treatment of cancer will be limited.

III. Harmful Effects of Radiation Therapy

Following the early enthusiastic development of ionizing radiation as an effective agent in shrinking and often ablating cancer, it became apparent that harmful side effects were associated with its use, generally manifested by acute and late damage of normal tissues, particularly the skin when lower energies of radiation were employed and deeper structures such as lung, brain, bone, kidney, etc. when more penetrating radiations became available.

Another effect was suspected clinically, beginning probably in the 1920s by some clinicians (Krebs, 1929): the enhancement of the spread and growth of tumour metastases by irradiation. These clinical impressions were confirmed experimentally by numerous independent investigators, although in some experimental animal tumour systems and radiation techniques the effect was not found. These findings involved radiations at sub-lethal levels of trans-planted and spontaneous tumours and, apparently through an entirely different mechanism, the heavy radiation of normal organs and tissues. These data will be presented and reviewed in order to attempt to establish the current concept of mechanisms and clinical significances.

A. *The Effect of Local Tumour Irradiation on Metastatic Behaviour*

Early experiments (Table I) indicated the enhancement of metastases

TABLE 1.

Effects of local tumour irradiation on metastatic behaviour

Year	Authors	Host	Tumour	Dose rads	Effect of radiation compared to non-irradiated control
1929	Krebs	mouse	sarcoma[a]	?	Slight increase of lung metastases. Inconclusive data.
1936	Yamamoto	rabbit	sarcoma[a]	?	Increase bone metastases. Inconclusive data.
1949	Kaplan and Murphy	mouse	mammary ca[a]	400–1000	Fourfold increase of pulmonary metastases.
1952	von Essen and Kaplan	mouse	mammary ca[a]	800–3000	Confirmed above. No effect following irradiation of host alone or tumour alone.
1953	Kaae	mouse	mammary ca	2000	Fourfold increase of pulmonary metastases.
1959a	Olch et al.	mouse	melanoma[a]	3000	Reduced numbers of pulmonary metastases in majority, increased numbers in remaining.
1959b					
1969	Fisher and Fisher	rats	Walker t.[a] and mamm. carc.[a]	1000–5000	No changes of metastatic frequency in Walker tumour. Increase of metastases in mamm. ca.
1970	Suit et al.	mouse	mammary ca[a]	6000–6400	Increased metastases in tumours not ablated.
1971	Van den Brenk and Sharpington	rat	sarcoma[a]	100–6000	Decreased metastases of primary treated early. Increased metastases if treated late.
1971	Crile and Deodhar	mouse	carcinoma[a]	4000	Decreased metastases in cured animals.
1972	Van den Brenk et al.	rat	sarcoma[a]	750–4000	Suggestive growth stimulation of metastases with 4000 rad to primary. No difference at this level between aerobic and anaerobic irradiation.
1973	Sheldon and Fowler	mouse	lympho-sarcoma[a]	1000	Increase of metastatic lymph node size.
1974	Sheldon et al.	mouse	sarcoma[a]	2000–5000 single and fractionated-range	Decreased metastases.
1974	Sheldon et al.	mouse	mammary ca[a]		Increase of metastases in non-cured radiated mice. Author state results inconclusive.
1975	Peters	mouse	squamous ca[a]	4500–6000	Improved survival with preop. radiation. Diminished survival with sub-lethal dose presumed due to increased metastases.
1976	McCredie et al.	mouse	fibrosarcoma	4000	No difference in lung metastases between irradiated and amputated tumours.

[a] Transplanted tumour.

following sub-lethal doses of radiation (Krebs, 1929; Yamamoto, 1936). However, these studies are considered inconclusive because of experimental conditions. In 1949, Kaplan and Murphy, following clinical observations of unusual widespread metastases of in-adequately irradiated squamous carcinoma of the lip and buccal mucosa, carried out laboratory investigations to determine whether this phenomenon existed, at least in inbred experimental animals. This result and those of several succeeding investigators (von Essen and Kaplan, 1952; Kaae, 1953; Fisher and Fisher, 1969) clearly confirmed that the rate of pulmonary metastases was increased in transplanted and spontaneous mammary carcinomas in inbred strains of mice and rats, following single exposure doses of radiation ranging from 400 to 3000 r. In the tumour systems tested there was a low (15%) to absent rate of spontaneous metastases while the rate of metastases following tumour irradiation was at least four times the spontaneous rate. The doses used were in no instances curative. In investigating the mechanisms of this phenomenon, von Essen and Kaplan (1952), determined that the effect was transient and involved *in situ* conditions. Their experiments tended to exclude the possibi-lities that irradiation of the host alone, i.e. in a non-tumour site, or the tumour *in vitro* with subsequent implantation were involved. By a process of exclusion it was considered that the phenomenon was transient and probably concerned facilitating the entry of tumour cells into blood vessels.

Subsequent investigations, employing other experimental animal tumour systems, have found a variety of responses including decreased, unchanged, and increased rates of metastases compared to untreated (or surgically treated) animals. For example, several (Van den Brenk and Sharpington, 1971; Crile, 1968; Sheldon *et al.*, 1974) found decreased rates of metastases (*see* Table 1). Van den Brenk and Sharpington noted that the metastatic rate was decreased if tumours were treated when quite small and were unlikely to have metasta-sised, while advanced tumours with a higher probability of metas-tasis had an enhanced growth of metastases following local tumour irradiation. Sheldon *et al.* (1974) noted that in mice with radiated tumours those with local cures had a low rate of metastasis while in those that were not cured a high rate of metastasis was noted even when the primary tumours were removed surgically. It is apparent from these and other experiments that a common factor in the observed phenomenon of increased metastatic rate following irra-diation is a dose of radiation insufficient to cure the primary lesion. In only a few instances was no effect on the metastatic frequency or size found following radiation therapy. Fisher and Fisher (1969) found no changes in pulmonary metastasis in the Walker tumour while a 38% frequency of lung metastases occurred in locally irradiated mammary carcinoma compared to nil in sham-irradiated mice. The primary tumour size of the irradiated mice was one-half of the sham-irradiated tumours at 80 days. McCredie *et al.* (1976) found no differences in metastasis whether the primary tumour was irradiated or amputated. No untreated controls were, however, included in that study.

It thus is apparent that in a variety of experimented animal tumour systems the effect of local tumour irradiations on the metastatic rate can be *stimulating, inhibiting*, or *absent*. It is not surprising that this should occur since the tumour-host relationship may vary widely in these systems and it is most likely that the effect of radiation is principally focused at the level of the local tumour and the tumour bed. It is unlikely from several experiments that systemic factors play a significant role. Van den Brenk and Sharpington (1971) postulated a growth stimulating substance released from sterile irradiated tumour cells to be involved in the accelerated growth of metastases from large, heavily irradiated tumours in an allogeneic rat sarcoma which metastasised rapidly and widely even when untreated. This effect could not be confirmed by Sheldon *et al.* (1974) studying a slow growing and late metastasising syngeneic mouse sarcoma system. The same authors state that their unresolved findings in the radiation of a transplanted mammary carcinoma (Sheldon *et al.*, 1974) with respect to enhanced metastasis following radiation, may be due to the more rapid tumour growth in irradiated control mice leading to death before the period of appearance of metastasis in treated mice. This discrepancy in life time available for appearance of metastases between treated and untreated animals may have been a factor in the experimental conditions of the earlier experiments (Kaplan and Murphy, 1949; von Essen and Kaplan, 1952; Kaae, 1953; Fisher and Fisher, 1969). However, von Essen and Kaplan (1952) attempted to correct this possible prejudicial condition by matched killing of mice in the experimental and control groups whenever a mouse became moribund or died. This technique confirmed Kaplan and Murphy's earlier experiments showing an enhancement of metastasis following radiation but not utilizing matched killing. However, another objection raised by Sheldon *et al.* (1974) concerns the discrepancy of tumour volumes in irradiated and unirradiated cases. They consider that the very large tumours in the unirradiated controls at the time of sacrifice could have caused greater "constitutional stress" and thus, presumably, inhibit the appearance of secondaries. In their critical evaluation of these time and volume factors in their own data they raise the following question: "A more pertinent question would be whether one would expect a metastasis incidence of 33% from recurrent tumours after irradiation when the incidence after curative irradiation is only 8%. In other words, do these data suggest that radiation itself, when not given in large enough doses to eradicate tumours, increases the risk of getting lung metastases?".

The presence of radiation inactivated tumour cells may result in growth of lethal tumours with 3 or 4 logs fewer viable tumour cells then without (Schnabel, 1975). A growth supporting capability of radiation inactivated tumour cells is a well-known phenomenon (Révész, 1956). Dead tumour cells can significantly increase the incidence of metastases of living tumour cells when they are injected simultaneously (Fidler, 1975). Morphological and biological alterations of irradiated cells have been described and related to an observed augmentation of metastases (Fisher and Fisher, 1969) It is still open to investigation whether admixture of radiation inactivated cells to viable cells leaving an irradiated primary tumour may be one of many possible mechanisms explaining observed increase of distant metastases in many experimental model systems.

This issue, therefore, remains controversial at the experimental level. In clinical radiation therapy the issue has been raised repeatedly (Krebs, 1929; Kaplan and Murphy, 1949; Stearns *et al.*, 1959) that certain irradiated tumours exhibit unusual patterns of metastasis generally when compared to surgical experience. All of these reports are anecdotal or even speculative. If, however, we accept to some extent, the evidence of well done-experiments with properly selected animal tumour systems as discussed by Scott (1972) then there should be concern about the consequences of non-curative radiation therapy in man. The conditions that may be of importance can be listed as follows:

(1) Inadequate radiation dose to ablate primary disease.
(2) Long time interval to surgery.
(3) Low rate of metastasis following effective therapy.

The use of planned pre-operative radiation therapy has not been associated with enhanced metastasis although Stearns (1959) noted a higher metastatic rate in a non-randomized series. Kraus and Perez-Mesa (1966) reported unusual metastatic spread of inadequately irradiated verrucous carcinomas of the oral cavity. However, they also considered that an anaplastic change had occurred in the histological patterns of these tumours. No such findings have been reported by investigators using experimental tumours.

In summary, a wide range of effects upon the rate and magnitude of metastasis occur following radiation therapy of a number of experimental animal tumour systems. In general metastasis appear to be enhanced in cases where non-curative doses are given and where "large" tumours are irradiated. Metastases are reduced when compared to untreated controls with curative radio-therapy and the treatment of "small" tumours. Experimental conditions of different tumour volume and different lethality of primary tumour growth in treated and untreated tumours render the interpretation of these results difficult with respect to mechanisms of action. The clinical significance of the phenomenon of enhanced metastasis following irradiation is not known. Suggestive evidence exists, however, that inadequate radiation may accelerate the spread of cancer and therefore further investigations are warranted to clearly define the import of this evidence.

B. *The Effects of Radiation of Normal Tissue Remote from Tumour on Metastatic Behaviour*

In contrast to the previously discussed effects of local tumour irradiation on metastasis frequency another phenomenon, apparently unrelated, was first noted by clinicians nearly 30 years ago and has been the subject of recent intensive investigation. This is the enhancement of metastatic spread into apparently normal tissues that have been previously irradiated. The tissues in question have generally been either the skin or lung. However, other organs have also been implicated. These observations have been made both in man with several well-documented examples and in experimental animal tumour systems.

Following the early reports by Schürch (1935) and Schwarz (1935) on the localization of metastases to heavily irradiated skin, the observations of Dao and Kovaric (1962) created an impact and generated a continuing controversy in the therapeutic oncology community. They studied patients with breast cancer who received surgery alone or post-operative radiation with orthovoltage techniques to the operated site which included the chest wall, axilla, supraclavicular area and, by transmission, the underlying lung. A

TABLE 2

Effects of normal tissue irradiation on metastatic behaviour

Year	Author	Host	Tumours	Irradiated tissue(s)	Dose rads	Effects on metastatic spread into irradiated normal tissue
1935	Schürch	man	gastric ca.	skin	?	Metastases confined to target tissue.
1935	Schwarz	man	breast ca.	skin	?	" " " "
1962	Dao and Kovaric	man	breast ca.	skin and lung	4500/3 weeks	Increased metastases in target tissue.
1963	Koike et al.	mouse	Ehrlich ascites[a]	liver	1500	Increased metastases.
1967a,b	Chu et al.	man	breast ca.	skin and lung		No increase.
1967	Dao and Yogo	rat	mamm. ca.[a]	lung	500–2000	Five fold increase with radiation prior to iv. inoculation.
1969	Fisher and Fisher	mouse	Walker tumour[a]	lung and liver	1000–2000	Increase size and number with radiation 1 to 7 days prior.
1970	Zeidman and Fidler	rabbit	V2 carcinoma[a]	whole body	400	Increased lung metastases with prior radiation.
1971	Cole and Halnan	man	breast ca.	skin	3500–4000 3–4 weeks	Four cases of metastases confined to target tissue.
1972	Fidler and Zeidman	rabbit	V2 carcinoma[a]	whole body	450	Increased radioisotope labelled tumour cells in irrad. tissue.
1973	Brown	mouse	KHT sarcoma[a]	lung	500–2000	Dose dependent enhancement disappearing after 3 weeks gap.
1973	Owen and Bostock	dog	melanoma + osteosarcoma	lung	1200	Reduction if radiation followed iv. injection or ablation. Enhancement in 4 cases where primary was not controlled.
1973	Van den Brenk et al.	rat	sarcoma[a]	lung, liver, kidney	1000–1500	Increased metastases with prior irradiation.
1973	Withers and Milas	mouse	fibrosarcoma[a]	lung	1000–3000	Ten-fold increase with prior irradiation.

Year	Author	Host	Tumours	Irradiated tissue(s)	Dose rads	Effects on metastatic spread into irradiated normal tissue
1974	Van der Brenk and Kelly	rats	Walker tumour[a]	lung	1250 (5 × 350)	Increased metastases; fractionated dose more effective than single dose.
1974	Vaage et al.	mouse	fibrosarcoma[a]	large volumes	300 to 1500	Volume dependent increased tumour growth outside target volume
1974b	Thompson	mouse	mamm. ca.[a]	lung	250–2000	Increased metastases: Effect seen with doses up to 9½ month gap. 1974.
1974	Peters	mouse	chondrosar-coma[a]	lung	1600–2000	Increased metastases with 5 week gap.
1975	Owen	dog	various	lung	600–1200	Increased metastases in 2 or 3 spont. tumours.
1976	Stjernswärd and Douglas	man	breast ca.	various sites	4000–4400	8 cases of metastases confined to target issue.

[a] Transplanted tumour.

unique observation was that a number of patients receiving post-operative radiation developed hundreds of metastases limited to the areas of skin that had been exposed to irradiation. They furthermore reported that the incidence of ipsilateral skin and lung metastases was considerably greater in patients receiving post-operative radiation therapy, than in those having surgery alone. Of importance in the interpretation of their data are the facts that the series was not the subject of a randomized trial and the clinical staging of patients receiving post-operative radiation therapy was generally more advanced; the technique of documenting the lung metastases was not described (radiation pulmonary fibrosis being considered a major differential finding); and an unusually high proportion of patients had severe and disabling radiation injuries, indicating radiation overdosage in many cases. Therefore the most significant conclusion that can be drawn from this and other clinical reports (*see* Table 2) is that a number of patients can be identified who demonstrate a selective distribution of metastases in the radiated skin which, in some instances at least, had a low probability of pre-existing tumour. This appears to be a rare phenomenon indeed as discussed by Chu *et al.* (1967a, b) and from numerous more recent reports on the results of radiation therapy in many sites and may be associated with exceptionally high doses of radiation sufficient to produce significant tissue damage. Thus the principal of *locus minoris resistentia* can be recalled and applied to the possibility that tissues damaged by irradiation to a certain extent can form a fertile locus for presumed circulating cancer cells which would otherwise be unlikely to survive and grow into clinically detectable metastases (Fisher and Fisher, 1975; Salsbury, 1975; Carter, 1976).

Following Dao and Kovaric's paper (1962) a series of experimental reports have confirmed the clinical observation that previously radiated tissues when exposed to blood-borne tumour cells will serve as a locus for implantation and pre-operative growth in contrast to non-irradiated tissues. This effect has been shown by several (Fisher and Fisher, 1969; Dao and Yogo, 1967; Brown, 1973a; Van den Brenk *et al.*, 1973) to require local tissue irradiation. Prior whole body irradiation alone was shown by Zeidman and Fidler (1970); Rosenau and Moon (1967) to enhance lung metastasis while others (Brown, 1973a) determined that shielding of the lung reduced the lung metastasis incidence to control levels. Several have shown that a local increased arrest of tumour cells in the lungs occurs whether the radiation is administered locally or to the total body (Withers and Milas, 1973; Fidler and Ziedman, 1972; Brown, 1973a).

It has been determined by several investigators that the phenomenon does not involve immune depression (Dao and Yogo, 1967; Van den Brenk et al., 1973), although Vaage et al. (1974) considered that suppression of tumour immune resistance factors may be operative if radiation is given shortly prior to tumour challenge. Others (Van den Brenk et al., 1973; Owen, 1975; Peters, 1974) considered that local tissue irradiation resulting in inflammatory changes including micro-thrombi in blood vessels and other local phenomena were primarily responsible for the enhanced implantation of circulating tumour cells.

In all experimental cases, radiation prior to challenge with injected tumour cells was necessary to demonstrate enhanced tumour take. This finding contrasts to earlier work by Vermund et al. (1956) who were able to inhibit the take of tumour fragments transplanted into heavily irradiated tissues.

Clinical implications have been carefully considered by Peters (1975) and Owen (1975). Both believe that there are significant experimental data to feel concerned about any programme of routine prophylactic wide field irradiation if there is a high probability of uncontrolled active tumour in the patient. If, on the other hand, there is reasonable evidence that the primary disease has been controlled, then there is considerable justification to prophylactically irradiated regional nodes at risk. This is certainly suggested by clinical evidence in the case of seminomas, rectal carcinoma (Roswit et al., 1970) and head and neck cancer (Lindberg and Jesse, 1968). On the other hand if there is a high risk of wide spread dissemination such as in breast cancer, Stjernswärd (1974) considers that "prophylactic" radiation following mastectomy enhances metastatic growth and shortens survival time.

It is now possible to delineate somewhat the mechanisms responsible for the phenomenon of enhanced tumour growth in previously irradiated tissue. The evidence as presented above indicates that a local as contrasted to a systemic effect is most likely. An increased entrapment or delayed release of cancer cell emboli in small vessels, probably blood vessels, has been demonstrated.

It has been shown (Hopewell, 1974; Reinhold and Buisman, 1975) that radiation of sufficient dosage can produce acute inflammatory changes in the fine vasculature including microthrombi, dilatation, and alteration of blood flow. It is conceivable that circulating tumour cells may be more easily trapped in these areas of local blockage. Van den Brenk et al. (1972) postulate another mechanism, a "feeder" effect of irradiated normal degenerating cells on implanted tumour cells involving a release of a growth stimulating substance. This is similar to the Révész effect (Révész, 1956) wherein survival and growth of tumour cells is enhanced by the proximity of sterile heavily irradiated cells. Thompson's data (1974) shows clearly that both metastasis frequency and the average volume of individual metastases were increased in radiated lungs. This tends to support the hypothesis of Van den Brenk *et al.* (1972) of a "feeder" effect. This phenomenon has been demonstrated to have latency periods following lung irradiation of periods from a few days up to $3\frac{1}{2}$ months and as long as $9\frac{1}{2}$ months (Thompson, 1974a, b). This time span seems certainly related to several different effects of radiation, since acute and clinic damage is encompassed in most mammalian systems during this period. Although several investigators (Brown, 1973a; Withers and Milas; 1973, Van den Brenk *et al.*, 1973; Van den Brenk and Kelly, 1974) noted that the period extended up to 42 days after radiation, Peters (1974) and Peters and Hewitt (1974) found an effect as late as 5 weeks and Thompson (1974) noted an effect at $9\frac{1}{2}$ months. This suggests that a curve of at least biphasic shape may be drawn describing the rise and fall of metastatic frequency with time following pulmonary radiation. The wide variety of tumour systems and doses utilized must, however, lend caution to this supposition.

The endothelium of many vessels contains activators of fibrinolytic activity as determined histochemically in biopsy specimens of the walls of epigastric superficial veins (Svanberg *et al.*, 1976). It has been proposed that the irradiation of a tumour damages its vessels which may help to inhibit its growth (Tomlinson, 1973). Irradiation damage to vessels in the periphery of the irradiation field may facilitate the nidation of circulating metastatic cells here and have the opposite effect leading to facilitation of tumour outgrowth.

Radiotherapy of the primary tumour in patients with osteogenic sarcoma has not improved survival. However, the finding from an ongoing trial with interferon therapy (Strander, 1976) may be relevant to the concept that radiotherapy as a localized form of treatment may have a general systemic effect. Thirteen cases of osteosarcomas without visible tumour left at the operation were treated weekly with Interferon for two years. There are 3 patients who have developed pulmonary metastasis and these are all in the group of patients who received full dose radiotherapy. In the patients operated only and treated with Interferon there has so far been no metastases, a positive and impressive result in itself. Out of the 13 patients 5 have local resection, 7 had amputation, and 9 of these patients has pre-operative radiotherapy. Our hypothesis may be that previous radiotherapy diminishes the positive effect of Interferon. However, it is too early to conclude this with so few observations, but the practical clinical implication of the finding is important enough to motivate it and to keep it under observation.

C. *Post-operative Irradiation and Secondary Spread in Breast Cancer*

Post-operative radiotherapy has documented therapeutical effects in controlling local regional recurrences (Montague and Nelson, 1975). It is clearly indicated in tumours that are known to have a high frequency of local regional spread and there is a low risk of disseminated disease. The problem and perhaps controversy starts in the forms of tumours where there is a high frequency of distant metastasis. Most forms of irradiation, independent of whether the thymus is in the target tissue or not, are known to induce a long lasting lymphopenia. There are clear animal experimental data that support the concept that a general immunosuppression will facilitate the outgrowth of micro-metastases. Again we are faced with the problem if we are going to believe results gained in experimental host systems and take them seriously clinically or if they are to be ignored.

Breast cancer offers a unique opportunity for analysing this question further (Stjernswärd, 1974) because of:

(1) One among many different biological parameters of breast cancer reflect immunological tumour host relationship in which the tumour antagonistic immune defence reactions of the host have been documented as cellular changes in the lymphoreticular system which are correlated with disease and survival characteristics.

(2) Prophylactic post operative adjuvant radiotherapy has a general systemic effect inducing a long lasting severe lympho-penia with various changes in the WBC cells sub-population. This in a situation where we have minimal residual disseminated disease in a high frequency.

(3) The high number of patients with breast cancer. Postulated immune surveillance mechanisms have, by definition, already failed in those patients who arrive with a manifest cancer. Any further effect of host anti-tumour immunities in such a situation must be judged realistically. Breast cancer being the most frequent tumour in women in most industrialized countries offers sufficiently high number of patients to hope to document even small differences.

Available controlled trials where the effect of pre- or post-operative radiotherapy can be evaluated have been analysed. An increased mortality in early breast cancer can be correlated to the routine use of local post-operative irradiations (Stjernswärd, 1974). Without any biological stratification the increased mortality varies between 1% and 10% in irradiated patients compared to those treated by operation alone. The mortality differences indicated in the trials analysed may be higher if histological lymph node negative patients were not included. Such patients were included in some of the trials. Such cases have a much lower risk of occult dissemination than those with histological positive lymph nodes. Radiotherapy-induced immune suppression will have no effect on the appearance of metastases and consequently on mortality in lymph node negative patients, where the probability of sub-clinical distant disease following surgery is very low. The same is also true for invalidating certain conclusions from a pre-operative irradiation therapy trial as discussed below. Furthermore, certain high risk groups may be identified, such as pre-menopausal women which demonstrated a distinctly higher risk of mortality when radiotherapy was included in their treatment.

The question whether the general immunosuppression caused by radiotherapy will lead to an acceleration of distant metastasis is a principal question not only for breast cancer, but for many other tumour forms. It cannot be excluded yet that the above observation may occur in other forms of tumours. However, the question is not yet settled and remains open, but breast cancer offers one of the most realistic tumour models in which to investigate this question. Besides the theoretical importance of these results throwing some light on the possible role of host immunity and postulated immune surveillance mechanisms in cancer patients, they also have a clear practical importance not without socio-economic value. It is important to separate the possible harmful effect of immunosuppression caused by radiotherapy from that of chemotherapy. Radiotherapy is a localized form of therapy with no effect on distant spread, while chemotherapy has a systemic anti-tumour effect. In the later situation a general immunosuppression will be positively balanced by the anti-tumour effect of the chemotherapy.

It is necessary to be critical of conclusions from certain controlled trials on the role of pre-operative radiotherapy and distant metastases when they state that there is "no effect of local irradiation on frequency of distant metastases" (de Schryver, 1975) when the trial as a matter of fact is not relevant for this question.

As noted earlier (Perez, 1970) patients with clinically localized, easily resectable lesions and/or with tumours where there is a high probability of clinically unrecognized metastases at the time of irradiation, will not be expected to benefit from pre-operative irradiation. Breast cancer Stage I and II would be such a group. In spite of this, clinical trials were done with pre-operative radiation in Stage I and II breast cancer stating that this form of radiotherapy has no effect on distant metastases (de Schryver, 1975). Furthermore, the local lymph node status is one of the most important prognostic indicators necessary for a proper biological stratification of patients, balancing the groups within a trial. Clinical evaluation, without histology, of lymph node status carries an error between 30% to 70%. When giving pre-operative radiotherapy the very important biological stratification criteria of lymph node status is not available. An unknown number of histological lymph node negative patients that are not balanced among the compared groups may thus be included: these breast cancer cases very likely have a lower risk of occult dissemination than those with positive nodes. Local radiotherapy may have no effect on the appearance of metastasis and consequently in mortality in such cases.

Results from most animal model systems suggest that irradiation of the primary tumour or the tumour host itself results in an increase of distant metastases. This raises the question whether we are to believe that animal models can give us useful clinical guidance or if we are prepared to disregard experimental results from animal models (Scott, 1972). Some few human data could support the experimental findings of increased total number and/or accelerated appearance of distant metastases after local irradiation of certain tumours, or after prophylactic post-operative irradiation of certain tissues.

IV. Summary

Radiation therapy has been shown to be a highly effective agent in the palliation of cancer metastases at many sites. These include lesions in bone, CNS, and skin. In addition, ionizing radiation plays a significant role in the curative treatment of acute leukemia with respect to the eradication of leukemia cells metastatic to the CNS. Utilizing principles based on the knowledge of cell killing kinetics an increasing role is seen for multi-modality therapy involving combinations of surgery, radiation, chemotherapy, and immunotherapy.

This can be visualized as a succession of treatments, each with specific roles in the progressive elimination of cancer cells from the body. Surgery is effective in removing a large bulk of tumour in a limited tissue volume; radiation therapy is effective in sterilizing a smaller number of tumour cells, perhaps up to 10^9, in a wider tissue volume, whereas systemic chemotherapy is useful in sterilizing small nests of remaining cells i.e. about 10^7 in the remaining portions of the body. Beyond this, immunotherapy in view of its low morbidity may have a role in eliminating the last remaining tumour cells from the body.

Thus the control of metastatic disease is primarily dependent on control of the primary site and secondarily dependent on the distribution and size of established metastatic foci. Radiation is a principal agent in control of localized and symptomatic metastases.

The possibly deleterious role of radiation therapy in cancer metastasis management has been reviewed: two distinct mechanisms have been identified; one, the apparent enhancement of metastases following radiation of the primary site; the other, the enhancement of metastases in normal tissues previously radiated.

In the first instance the data are entirely developed in experimental animal-tumour systems; the findings vary among the systems from enhancement to suppression of metastases. The factors that appear to be causally related are doses of radiation incapable of total sterilization and tumours that are large and have a finite but low metastasis rate when not treated. The clinical significance of these findings is not established.

In contrast the second phenomenon, that of metastasis enhancement in previously irradiated tissues is a generally consistent finding both experimentally and clinically. It varies considerably with tumour type, radiated site, radiation dose, volume, and interim period.

The mechanisms of both these phenomena are not established but may well involve microvascular injury. Radiotherapists should be well aware of these phenomena when embarking on new ventures in methodology.

References

Ainsfield, F. J. (1976). *JAMA*, **235** (1), 67–75.

Almgard, L. E., Edsmyr, F. and Franzen, S. (1970). *Läkartidningen*, **69**, 153–167.

Bloom, H. J. G., Wallace, E. N. K. and Henk, J. M. (1969). *Amer. J. Roentg. Radium Therapy Nuccl. Med.* **15**, 43–62.

Brown, J. M. (1973a). *Br. J. Cancer*, **46**, 613–618.
Brown, J. M. (1973b). *Cancer Res.* **33**, 1217–1224.
Campbell, A. C., Hersey, P., MacLennan, I. C. M., Kay, H. E. M. and Pike, M. C. (1973). *Brit. Med. J.* **2**, 385–388.
Carter, R. L. (1976). "Scientific Foundation of Oncology" (T. Symington and R. L. Carter, eds), pp. 172–180. William Heinemann Medical Books Ltd., London.
Chu, F. C., Lucas, J. C. and Farrow, J. H. (1967a). *Amer. J. Roentg.* **99**, 987–994.
Chu, F. C., Nisce, C., Baker, A. S., Sattar, A. and Laughlin, J. S. (1967b). *Radiology*, **89**, 216–223.
Cole, H. and Halnan, K. E. (1971). *Clin. Radiol.* 133–135.
Crile, G., Jr. (1968). *Surg. Gynecol. & Obstet.* **126**, 1270–1272.
Crile, G., Jr. and Deodhar, S. D. (1971). *Cancer*, **27**, 629–634.
Dao, Th. L. and Yogo, H. (1967). *Cancer*, **20**, 2020–2024.
Dao, Th. L. and Kovaric, J. (1962). *Surgery*, **52**, 203–212.
Dische, S. (1976). Personal communications.
von Essen, C. F. (1963). *Radiology*, **81**, 881–883.
von Essen, C. F. and Kaplan, H. S. (1952). *J. Nat. Cancer Inst.* **12**, 883–892.
Evans, A. E. (1975). *Cancer*, **35**, 48–54.
Fidler, I. J. (1975). *Radiation Onc. Biol. Phys.* **1**, 93–96.
Fidler, I. J. and Zeidman, I. (1972). *J. Med.* **3**, 172–177.
Fisher, B. and Collins, V. (1968). In "Cancer Therapy by Integrated Radiation and Operation" (Rush and Greenlaw, eds), pp. 28–33. Thomas, Springfield.
Fisher, E. R. and Fisher, B. (1969). *Cancer*, **24**, 39–55.
Fisher, E. R. and Fisher, B. (1975). *Int. J. Rad. Onc. Biol. Phys.* **1**, 87–91.
Fitzpatrick, P. J. and Rider, W. D. (1976). *Int. J. Rad. Onc. Biol. Phys.* **1**, 197–207.
Fletcher, G. H. (1973). "Textbook of Radiotherapy", pp. 816, 2nd edn. Lea & Febiger, Philadelphia.
Ghavimi, F., Exelby, P. R., D'Angio, G. J., Cham, W., Lieberman, P. H., Tan, C., Miké, V. and Murphy, M. L. (1975). *Cancer*, **35**, 677–686.
Goldie, J., Rosengren, B., Moberg, E. and Hedelin, E. (1970). *Acta Radiologica Therapy Physics Biol.* **9**, 311–322.
Hall, T. C. (1976). *Cancer suppl.* **23**, No. 2, 1218–1225.
Halnan, K. E. (1975). Proc. XI Int. Cancer Congress Florence 1974, Vol. 5, pp. 181–186. Excerpta Medica, Amsterdam.
Henderson, E. S. (1973). In "Cancer Medicine" (J. F. Holland and E. Frei III, eds), pp. 1173–1199. Lea & Febiger, Philadelphia.
Higgins, G. A., Dwight, R. W. (1972). *Surg. Clin. North. Am.* **52**, 847.
Hopewell, J. W. (1974). *Brit. J. Radiol.*, **47**, 157–158.
Hustu, H. O., Aur, R. J. A., Verzosa, M. S., Simone, J. V. and Pinkel, D. (1973). *Cancer*, **32**, 585–597.
Johnson, R. J. R. (1965). "Gynecological Cancer Treated with Cobalt under Hyperbaric Conditions in Hyperbaric Oxygen and Radiation Therapy of Cancer (J. M. Vcath, ed), pp. 185–206. McCutcheam Publishing Co., Berkeley, Calif., USA.
Johnson, R. E. (1975). *Cancer*, **35**, 242–246.
Johnson, R. E. (1976). *Radiology*, **86**, 1085–1089.
Kaae, S. (1953). Metastatic Frequency of Spontaneous Mammary Carcinomas in Mice Following Biopsy and Following Local Roentgen Irradiation.
Kaplan, H. S. and Murphy, E. D. (1949). *J. Nat. Cancer Inst.* **9**, 407–413.
Koike, A., Nakazato, H. and Moore, G. E. (1963). *Cancer*, **16**, 716–720.

Kraus, F. T. and Perez-Mesa, C. (1966). *Cancer,* **19**, 26–38.

Krebs, C. (1929). *Acta Radiol., Suppl.* **8**, 1–133.

Lindberg, R. D. and Jesse, R. H. (1968). *Amer. J. Roentgen.* **102**, 132–137.

Loeffler, R. K. and Puterbaugh, M. R. (1975). *Amer. J. Roentgen.* **123**, 170–178.

MacLennan, I. C. M., Kay, H. E. M., Festenstein, M., Smith, P. G. and Medical Research Council's Working Party on Leukemia in Childhood (1976). *Br. J. Haematol.* (in press).

McCredie, J. A., Inch, W. R. and Cowie, H. C. (1976). *Cancer,* **31**, 983–987.

Medical Research Council Report by Working Party on Leukemia in Childhood (1975). *Brit. Med. J.,* 563–566.

Medical Research Council (1973). *Brit. Med. J.* **2**, 381–384.

Montague, E. D. and Nelson, A. J. III (1975). Vol. 6 Proc. XI Int. Cancer Congress, Florence 1974, pp. 43–53. Excerpta Medica, Amsterdam.

Nissen-Meyer, R. (1975). Vol. 6 Proc. XI Int. Cancer Congress, Florence 1974, pp. 25–32. Excerpta Medica, Amsterdam.

Olch, P. D., Eck, R. V. and Smith, R. R. (1959a). *Cancer Res.* **19**, 464–467.

Olch, P. D., Eck, R. V. and Smith, R. R. (1959b). *Cancer,* **12**, 23–26.

Order, S. E., Hellman, S., von Essen, C. F. and Kligerman, M. M. (1968). *Radiology,* **91** (1), 149–153.

Owen, L. (1975). *Europ. J. Cancer,* **11**, 35–36.

Owen, L. N. and Bostock, D. E. (1973). *Europ. J. Cancer,* **9**, 747–752.

Perez, C. A. (1970). *Front. Rad. Therapy Onc.* **5**, 1–29.

Peters, L. J. and Hewitt, H. B. (1974). *Br. J. Cancer,* **29**, 279–291.

Peters, L. J. (1974). *Br. J. Radiol.* **47**, 827–829 (letter).

Peters, L. J. (1975a). *Br. J. Cancer,* **31**, 293–300.

Peters, L. J. (1975b). *Br. J. Cancer,* **32**, 355–372.

Potter, J. F. (1975). *Cancer,* **35**, 84–90.

del Regato, J. A. (1974). *Amer. J. Roentgenol.* **120**, 504–520.

Reinhold, H. S. and Buisman, G. H. (1975). *Br. J. Radiol.* **48**, 727–731.

Révész, L. (1956). *Nature,* **178**, 1391–1392.

Riches, E. W. (1968). *JAMA,* **204**, 230–231.

Rosen, G., Wollner, N., Tan, C., Wu, S. J., Hadju, S. I., Cham, V., D'Angio, G. J. and Murphy, M. L. (1974). *Cancer,* **33**, 384–393.

Rosenau, W. and Moon, H. D. (1967). *Cancer Res.* **27**, Part I, 1973–1981.

Roswit, B., Higgins, G. A., Shields, W. and Keehn, R. J. (1970). *Front. Rad. Therapy Onc.* **5**, 163.

Salsbury, A. J. (1975). *Cancer Treatment Review,* **2**, 55–72.

Schnabel, F. M. (1975). *Cancer,* **35**, 15–24.

de Schryver, A. (1975). *Bull. Cancer,* **62**, 175–182.

Schürch, O. (1935). *Zeitschr. für Krebsforschung,* **41**, 47–50.

Schwarz, G. (1935). Strahlentherapie, **53**, 674–681.

Scott, O. (1972). *Brit. Med. Bull.* **29**, 59–62.

Serrou, B., Dubois, J. B. and Serre, A. (1975). *Biomedicine,* **23**, No. 6, 236–240.

Sheldon, P. W. (1974). *Br. J. Cancer,* **30**, 416–420.

Sheldon, P. W. and Fowler, J. F. (1973). *Br. J. Cancer,* **28**, 508–514.

Sheldon, P. W., Begg, A. C., Fowler, J. F. and Lansley, I. F. (1974). *Br. J. Cancer,* **30**, 342–348.

Simone, J. V., Aur, J. A. R., Hustu, H. O., Verzosa, M. and Pinkel, D. (1975). *Cancer,* **35**, 25–35.

Stearns, M. W., Jr., Deddish, M. R. and Quan, S. H. (1959). *Surg. Gynecol. & Obstet.* **109**, 225–229.

Stein, J. J. (1973). *Front. Radiation Ther. Onc.* **8**, 18–25.

Stjernswärd, J. (1974). *Lancet*, **2**, 1285–1286.

Stjernswärd, J. (1975). Vol. 6 Proc. XI Int. Cancer Congress, Florence 1974. Excerpta Medica, Amsterdam, Vol. 6, 38–42.

Stjernswärd, J. and Douglas, P. (1976). *In* "Cancer Invasion and Metastasis: Biologic Mechanisms and Therapy" (S. B. Day *et al.* eds) pp. 311–323. Raven Press, New York.

Strander, H. (1976). Personal communication.

Strong, E. W., Henschke, U. K., Nickson, J. J., Frazell, E. L., Tollefsen, H. R. and Hilaris, B. S. (1966). *Cancer*, **10**, 509–516.

Suit, H. D. and Kastelan, A. (1970. *Cancer*, **26**, 232–238.

Suit, H. D., Sedlacek, R. S. and Gilette, E. L. (1970). *Radiology*, **95**, 189–194.

Suit, H. D., Russel, W. O. and Martin, R. G. (1973). *Cancer*, **31**, 1247–1255.

Suit, H. (1973). *In* "Textbook of Radiotherapy" (G. H. Fletcher, ed), pp. 75–121, 2nd edn. Lea & Febiger, Philadelphia.

Svanberg, L., Astedt, B. and Kullander, S. (1976). *Acta Obst. Gynecol. Scand.* **55**, 49–51.

Thomas, E. D., Buckner, C. D., Clif, R. A. *et al.* (1973). *Transpl. Proc.* **5**, 917–922.

Thompson, S. C. (1974a). *Br. J. Cancer*, **30**, 332–336.

Thompson, S. C. (1974b). *Br. J. Cancer*, **30**, 337–341.

Tomlinson, R. H. (1973). *Brit. Med. Bull.* **29**, 29–32.

Tubiana, M. (1976). Personal communication.

Vaage, J., Doroshow, J. H. and DuBois, T. T. (1974). *Cancer Res.* **34**, 129–137.

Van den Brenk, H. A. S. and Sharpington, C. (1971). *Br. J. Cancer*, **25**, 812–830.

Van den Brenk, H. A. S. and Kelly, H. (1974). *Br. J. Cancer*, **28**, 349–353.

Van den Brenk, H. A. S., Burch, W. M., Orton, C. and Sharpington, C. (1973). *Br. J. Cancer*, **27**, 291–306.

Van den Brenk, H. A. S., Moore, V., Sharpington, C. and Orton, C. (1972). *Br. J. Cancer*, **26**, 402–412.

Vermund, H. *et al.* (1956). *Radiation Res.* **5**, 354–364.

Withers, H. R. and Milas, L. (1973). *Cancer Res.* **33**, 1931–1936.

Zeidman, I. and Fidler, I. J. (1970). *J. Med.* **1**, 9–14.

Yamamoto, T. (1936). *J. Obstet. & Gynecol.* **19**, 559–569

Chapter IV

Chemotherapy of Experimental Metastasis

FEDERICO SPREAFICO AND SILVIO GARATTINI*

Istituto di Ricerche Farmacologiche "Mario Negri" Via Eritrea 62, 20157 Milano, Italy

I. Introduction

There appears to exist today little ground for disputing the conclusion that principles of chemotherapeutic intervention developed in experimental model systems have played a crucial role in bringing about the substantial advances in the cure rates of several human neoplastic conditions obtained in recent years. Although cognizant of the importance of the introduction to the clinic of a larger number of effective antitumour drugs, we surmise that the chief factor in current greater therapeutical possibilities and achievements relative to the past has been the exploitation of available agents along more rational lines which, in many respects, represent the transfer to man of philosophies first developed and tested at the animal level. In this search for always more effective antineoplastic chemotherapeutic treatments, two historical phases could be recognized. The first has essentially employed fast-growing animal neoplasms, such as the leukaemia-lymphomas, with treatments given early after tumour transplantation. More recently, the emphasis has shifted to the treatment, or attempts thereto, of solid and more

* Supported by NCI grant PHRB 1 ROI CA 12764 and CNR contract No. 75.00569.04

advanced tumours, i.e. of experimental models of those clinical conditions which pose at the present time, the greatest therapeutic difficulties. The centring of the attention of experimental oncologists to the specific problem of metastasis treatment and/or prevention, is thus only relatively recent. In a volume of this type, the clinical importance of metastasis needs not to be emphasized since it is common knowledge that, except in inoperable cases, death of the patient with a malignancy only rarely results from the primary tumour growth or its local recurrence, but almost invariably the patient succumbs to metastatic disease.

In this chapter we will briefly consider three general and interrelated aspects which, we believe, are basic for the development of more effective anti-metastatic treatments. Specifically, we will discuss firstly, some principles evolved at the experimental animal level and which appear as especially relevant for metastasis inhibition by adjuvant chemotherapy; secondly, the problem of representative animal model systems for the investigation of cancerous dissemination and metastasis formation will be considered; and lastly, the possibilities of alternative approaches to anti-metastasis treatment not relying exclusively on classical chemotherapy will be examined.

II. Some Basic Chemotherapeutic Principles for Metastasis Treatment

A number of basic principles evolved over the years in experimental cancer chemotherapy appear to bear special relevance for guiding towards more rationalized anti-metastatic interventions employing the classical therapeutic modalities of surgery and/or radiotherapy and chemotherapy. As is true for primary tumours, and also for neoplastic secondaries, one can theoretically divide the total malignant population into three compartments; specifically, one composed of the actively replicating cells; a second comprising those elements temporarily non-dividing but potentially capable of replication; and thirdly, that containing the cells which have completely lost their capacity to multiply and whose destiny is cell death or loss from the neoplastic mass. It is generally accepted that the growth curve of animal cancers (and presumably human cancers as well) follows a Gömpertzian function, i.e. a curve in which growth is at every instant exponential but with a growth constant which is simultaneously exponentially retarded. In other words, this means that as the neoplasm increases in size, its mass doubling time becomes progressively longer. However, malignant growth is recognizable as clearly Gömpertzian when the tumour is measured over its palpable, clinically measurable range, whereas for smaller number of cells (1 to 10^7–10^8), i.e. in the clinically indetectable period, an exponential or near exponential growth curve is seen; a point which has some practical implications for the clinician whose aim is curative treatment of disseminated neoplasms. The Gömpertzian behaviour of malignant growths in their clinically apparent period is attributable to the interplay of at least three factors; namely, the increase in the average generation time of actively multiplying cells, as directly proven in several solid and lymphomatous animal tumours (Wilcox et al., 1965; Yankee et al., 1967; Schabel, 1969a; Tannock, 1969; Simpson-Herren et al., 1974), a progressively increasing cell loss from the neoplasm because of cell death and/or cell shedding and, lastly, the increase in the proportion of cells entering the temporarily non-replicating compartment, i.e. following a common nomenclature, showing Type II Resistance.* In parallel, a reduction of the tumour mass whether obtained by chemotherapy or by retransplantation of fragments to a new host, brings about a shortening in the mass doubling time, which is most probably the consequence of both a reduction in the average generation of time of proliferating elements and of an increase in the growth fraction of the tumour, i.e. of the proportion of the cells in proliferation. That the reduction in size entails shortening of the average cell generation time has been demonstrated not only in experimental (Schabel, 1975a) but also for human malignancies as varied as ovarian cancer (Sheehy et al., 1974) and acute lymphocytic leukaemia (Karle et al., 1973). Because of its direct relevance to this discussion, a clear illustration of the different cytokinetic parameters of the primary, palpable Lewis lung carcinoma (a mainstay in experimental metastasis investigations) and of its pulmonary micrometastases is presented by the data of Table 1 in which are also shown for reference purposes the same values for a few "standard" experimental tumours. The conclusion that the smaller the neoplastic mass the higher its doubling capacity, has obvious therapeutic consequences, since the latter dictates the level of sensitivity to drugs inhibiting cellular multiplication. The larger percentage of metabolically active cells will, in fact, increase the sensitivity of the neoplastic population to cell cycle-specific agents and this has been directly demonstrated with Arabinosylcytosine

---

* Those cells which fail to undergo DNA replication during effective drug exposure, or after exposure but prior to DNA repair.

TABLE 1

Tumour growth rates and cytokinetic parameters in animal tumours

Tumour	Tumour mass (mg) or cell no. at time of study	Measured doubling time (days)	Calculated % growth fraction	Cell loss factor (%)	Pulse labelling index (%)	Calculated mode and (range) of intermitotic times (hr)
L 1210 i.p.	10^6	0·5	82–100	0	65	11 (8–18)
	10^8–10^9		69		53	15 (5–28)
Ehrlich ascites i.p.	10^7	0·5	90	0	69	15 (9–20)
	10^8	6·0	43	0	25	75 (30– >42)
3LL primary s.c.	300	2·5	84	65	55	18 (8– >40)
	4200	9·6	51	78	28	24 (8– >50)
3LL metast. lung	microscopic	2·3	61 or >	57 or >	37 or >	15 (8– >40)
B16 s.c.	34	1·3	36	0	26	12 (5–40)
	560	1·9			16	19 (8– >50)

From Skipper, 1974.

(Griswold *et al.*, 1970). In addition, it should be recalled that for a number of non-cell cycle-specific cancer chemotherapeutic agents also, the cell killing efficacy is higher on proliferating than on resting cells (Valeriote and Van Putten, 1975). This reasoning leads thus to a first set of conclusions of direct clinical relevance. Firstly, metastasis are to be expected to be more sensitive to chemotherapy in general, and to cell cycle-specific agents in particular, than the primary tumour from which they are derived and the smaller the size of the secondary outgrowth the higher this differential sensitivity will be. Secondly, the insensitivity of a primary tumour to a given chemotherapeutic treatment does not necessarily predict the response of its metastases to the same regimen. Thus even those solid advanced tumours which had limited response to chemotherapy alone may fare much better in the context of a combined surgery-chemotherapy modality. It has also to be concluded that the treatment scheduling for an effective anti-metastatic inhibition should take into account this differential cell population kinetics. Directly connected with the last point above is another frequently overlooked but practically important tenet clearly established experimentally, namely that 50 or 30% reduction in tumour mass may actually represent more than 50 or 30% tumour cell kill. This point, which was firstly pointed out by Wilcox *et al.* (1965) has recently been clearly re-demonstrated by Steel and Adams (1975) showing that doses of Cyclophosphamide which induce an approximately 50% regression of primary 3LL masses with a nadir at 7–8 days, actually produced an approximately 5 log (i.e. 99,999%) tumour stem cell kill at 3 hr after drug injection. Multiplication of the "spared" cells and lysis of the killed elements, the two constantly changing and opposite factors whose integration determines tumour volume modifications, have different rates; thus the nadir of regression is delayed in comparison to the time of maximal cell destruction. Consequently, tumour cell kill after effective but non-curative chemotherapy of large neoplastic masses may be underestimated; the implications of this fact for effective drug scheduling and for expressing objective judgments on chemotherapy potential need not be belaboured.

Most of the statements so far advanced centre on the true basic law of cancer chemotherapy, namely that the "curability" of neoplasms is dependent on the number of viable neoplastic cells present in the body at the start of chemotherapy. This conclusion which is valid for all experimental tumours investigated and is very succinctly illustrated by the data of Table 2, together with its corollary that the "curability" of cancer by surgery (and/or radiation) is related to the

TABLE 2

Relationship between tumour burden and curability with chemotherapy in the i.m. Lewis lung carcinoma

Days after trans-plant	Approx. primary tumour weight (g)	metast.	Cyclo-P (mg/kg)				Me CCNU (mg/kg)			
			300		200		25		15	
			% cures	% ILS	% cures	% ILS	% cures	% ILS	% cures	% ILS
5	$\simeq 0.1$	—	60	115	45	65	30	105	0	55
10	0.5	+	10	60	0	30	0	60	0	20
15	2	+	0	35	0	0	0	25	—	—

ILS = increase in lifespan; Cyclo-P = cyclophosphamide; Me CCNU = methyl CCNU (NSC 95441); tumour inoculum: 2×10^5 cells i.m.

extent of dissemination at the start of these therapies, represents the cornerstone of a logical approach to the treatment of metastasis.

In addition to the reasons mentioned above for explaining the inverse relationship between sensitivity to chemotherapy and the tumour burden, and which have essentially dealt with Type II Resistance, two further factors have to be considered. The first consists in the fact that the larger the total malignant mass, e.g. the higher the number of tumour cells, progressively higher will be the proportion of the permanently drug-resistant variants,* which have been estimated to be one in 10^6–10^7 tumour cells in the case of single drug resistance (Hutchison and Schmid, 1973 and DeWys, 1973). On the basis of presently available animal data recently submitted to extensive analysis by Skipper (1974), the conclusion can be advanced that drug-resistant cells are, if not the principal, a major mechanism of failure following single drug chemotherapy in those neoplastic conditions (leukaemias as well as solid tumours) which at the beginning of treatment have a burden above 10^6–10^7 cells and which show an initial good response to chemotherapy. It should be noted that with such "good responder" tumours no especially extensive treatment in terms of courses or drug doses is necessary before observing the appearance of a neoplastic population showing a significant or total resistance to the drug which selected it. Five–six doses of Cyclophosphamide are capable of inducing significant resistance in L 1210 leukaemia cells (Hutchison and Schmid, 1973) and data of Schabel and his group (cited by Skipper, 1974) support

* The so-called type I Resistance.

the conclusion that in solid metastasising murine tumours as Lewis lung (3LL) carcinoma or B16 melanoma, even as few as 2–3 doses of an highly effective agent as Methyl-CCNU may be sufficient to select a resistant cell population. Type II Resistance is, on the other hand, the principal basis for the failure of chemotherapy in those large, solid neoplasms whose response to chemotherapy is poor even at the beginning of treatment.

The third factor, that in addition to "resting" cells and resistant variants, can explain the relationship between tumour burden and its sensitivity to chemotherapy, is represented by the increasing probability for the establishment of architectural or anatomical sanctuaries (Type III Resistance). With greater tumour masses or higher cell numbers, higher chances will exist for the existence of sites either within the tumour or in selected organs, where malignant cells will be protected from efficient exposure to cytotoxic compounds. In this connection one recent type of observation is worthwhile recalling for its possible synergism with previously mentioned mechanisms in giving a comparatively greater responsiveness of metastasis to chemotherapy. We refer to the finding that chemotherapeutic agents may accumulate in metastatic outgrowths in greater amounts than in the respective primary animal tumour This preferential distribution was initially noted for 6-Mercaptopurine and Methotrexate in the Sarcoma 180 lymph nodal metastases developing after intratibial tumour transplantation in mice and has successively been confirmed for Adriamycin and Daunomycin in the pulmonary secondaries of the 3LL carcinoma (Donelli and Spreafico, 1976) as shown in Table 3, which shows the integrated drug concentration per time values calculated per unit mass. Some recent data of Steel and Adams (1975) showing 10 times greater killing of neoplastic stem cells in the pulmonary metastasis than in the primary 3LL tumour after Cyclophosphamide, a cell cycle non-specific agent, probably have their explanation in this better drug delivery through a "better" tumour microvasculature. The latter also plays a role in the markedly lower hypoxic fraction (a major determinant of radiotherapeutic effectiveness) of the lung nodules as compared to the primary tumour seen in the same and other neoplastic systems (Suit and Maeda, 1967; Shipley et al., 1975).

A detailed review of the wealth of experimental data (see for instance Griswold et al., 1968; Humphreys and Karrer, 1970; Mayo et al., 1972; Schabel 1975a,b) which has led to the formulation of the conclusions very briefly presented above, would be impossible in a chapter of this length; we have therefore chosen from our experience a restricted series of results which can be representative of the major points so far touched on (Tables 4 and 5). We have also purposely omitted from this discussion, immunotherapy as an antimetastatic

TABLE 3

Adriamycin and Daunomycin levels in the primary i.m. Lewis lung carcinoma and its metastasis

Tissue	Drug	Drug equiv. (μg/g) at time						c × t (24 hr)
		15 min	30 min	60 min	8 hr	24 hr	72 hr	
Primary i.m. tumour	Adria.	3·9 ± 2·4	6·5 ± 0·4	7·0 ± 0·5	5·8 ± 0·2	5·6 ± 0·9	4·8 ± 0·5	8,940 ± 815
	Dauno.	2·0 ± 0·2	2·4 ± 0·3	1·9 ± 0·3	2·8 ± 0·5	1·9 ± 0·3	1	3,520 ± 595
Lung metast.	Adria.	19·0 ± 3·6	20·5 ± 0·4	18·6 ± 3·0	11·0 ± 1·1	9·3 ± 1·5	5·1 ± 1·1	17,215 ± 2,030
	Dauno.	20·3 ± 3·7	30·2 ± 2·1	15·7 ± 2·4	13·6 ± 1·4	10·8 ± 1·3	3·2 ± 0·6	19,320 ± 2,240

Drugs (15 mg/kg i.v.) were injected 25 days after the i.m. transplant of $2 \cdot 10^5$ tumour cells.

TABLE 4

Curability by surgery-chemotherapy in the Lewis lung carcinoma system: influence of disease stage

Day after transplant	Approx. primary tumour weight (g)	Metast.	% cures and (% ILS)				
			Surgery	MeCCNU (×1)	MeCCNU (×2)	Surgery + MeCCNU (×1)	Surgery + MeCCNU (×2)
9	0·3	+	0	5 (70)	10 (60)	30 (80)	30 (125)
14	1·8	+	0	0 (35)	0 (50)	10 (65)	30 (55)

Dose of MeCCNU was 25 mg/kg i.p. and the interval 7 days.

TABLE 5

Curability by surgery-chemotherapy in the Lewis lung carcinoma system: influence of disease stage

Day after transplant	Approx. primary tumour weight (g)	Metast.	% cures and (% ILS)			
			Surgery	Cyclo-P	Surgery + Cyclo-P	Surgery + Cyclo-P + MeCCNU
9	0·3	+	0	0 (45)	25 (90)	70 (245)
14	1·8	+	0	0 (10)	0 (55)	20 (160)
18	3·5	+	0	0 (0)	0 (20)	—

Cyclo-P dose was 150 mg/kg i.p. and for MeCCNU 25 mg/kg i.p.

approach; this decision was made since this type of treatment is considered in *Chapter VI*.

From what was briefly discussed above, the obvious conclusion can thus be drawn that, considering only classical treatment modalities, the most effective approach to the cure of relatively large, solid experimental malignancies which have metastasised, is represented by the initial reduction of total neoplastic burden through surgery (and/or radiation) of the primary followed by chemotherapy of the micrometastases. It also becomes clear that a delay of treatment until neoplastic secondaries have become clinically detectable (i.e. have reached the number of 10^9 cells or more,*) will be met with

* Assuming a mean cell diameter of 15 microns, the number of tumour cells in micrometastases of 1, 5 and 10 mm in diameter, can be estimated to be $3·0 \times 10^5$, $3·7 \times 10^7$ and $3·0 \times 10^8$ cells, respectively. With a cell diameter of 10 microns, the respective estimates are $1·0 \times 10^6$, $1·3 \times 10^8$ and $1·0 \times 10^9$ cells.

significantly lower chances of being "curative" (indeed, of being more than marginally effective) since chemotherapy that may be capable of destroying limited tumour burdens will be ineffective in the face of 10^9 or more such cells.

The value of combination chemotherapy employing non-cross-resistant agents appears now unquestionable at the clinical level also; accordingly its benefits in addition for the eradication of metastases do not need to be especially emphasized; the data of Table 5 may be representative in this respect. Optimal two-drug combinations may result in 10–100 times greater cell kill than that obtainable with the single agents used at the maximally tolerated doses. However, given the first order kinetics* followed by cytotoxic agents in their inactivation of tumour cells, such seemingly limited extra cell killing may indeed represent the crossing of the line between tumour progression and regression, i.e. curability. It has also to be noted that for only a minority of two drug-combinations the resulting toxicity has been of a synergistic type, whereas for the majority it has been additive, lower than additive or even non-additive also in man (Frei, 1972).

Attention has been called repeatedly in the preceding sections to the crucial role played by the tumour burden at the beginning of treatment in determining the final outcome of cancer chemotherapy. The possibility of estimating metastatic spreading at the time of first diagnosis and surgical intervention, i.e. the dimension of the cell kill required in a population of cancerous patients, is thus a focal point in guiding towards more rationalized answers to questions such as: is further treatment beyond surgical removal of the primary outgrowth necessary? If so, what kind of treatment is advised and for how long? Reasonably accurate estimates of metastatic burden, or of the therapeutically more important residual tumour burden after primary resection, can and have been obtained for a number of experimental neoplasms. Assuming that 1 g of neoplastic tissue corresponds to 10^9 cells, the curve of metastatic growth in the lungs after the i.m. transplant of 2×10^5 3LL carcinoma cells in C57Bl/6 mice is shown in Fig. 1.

On the assumption that the period to tumour recurrence is directly related to the number of viable cells which have escaped surgery (or radiotherapy) of the primary, a fact easily proven in experimental tumours of various types, it is then possible to obtain estimates of the metastatic tumour extension present at diagnosis for human neoplastic conditions also. In a provocative series of reports, Skipper (1974,

---

* I.e. when acting on a metabolically homogenous population, a constant effective dose will kill a constant fraction, and not number, of cells, irrespective of neoplasm size.

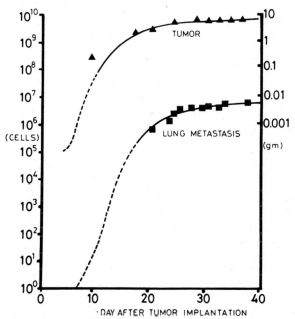

Fig. 1. Growth curves for the primary intramuscular Lewis lung carcinoma and its lung metastasis in C57B1/6 mice

1975) has produced such an analysis for common human malignancies such as breast carcinoma and osteogenic sarcoma. Relating clinically observed recurrence rates after surgery, available data on the overall median doubling times of small metastatic lesions (i.e. 30–40 days) and assuming that the limit to clinical detection of a recurrence is 10^9 cells (corresponding to a spherical mass 10 mm in diameter) and exponential growth until this size, then the calculated median residual burdens for various types of mammary carcinoma patients are presented in Table 6. Following the same principles, the calculated frequency distribution of patients with different residual cell numbers of osteogenic sarcoma, a tumour for which the overall median doubling time of metastatic cells is 10–20 days, are given in Table 7. It is obvious that these are rough estimates, since median values were considered and the ranges for the doubling times are known to be large.* However, these estimates have the value of

* Wider ranges in recurrence rates can be expected to occur when very low residual cells are present, since the probability will be higher for the chance selection of cells having "slower than median" overall doubling time which will not be overgrown by those elements with the median reproductive rate capacity. Evidence for such cellular variability in doubling time capacity is clear for animal tumours, and may provide an explanation for very late recurrences (after 10 years) observed in man after resection of certain primaries; the possibility of an activation of "dormant" disseminated cells cannot be dismissed, however.

TABLE 6

Estimates of residual tumour burden in mammary cancer patients after surgery assuming overall doubling times for metastatic cells of 30 or 40 days

Viable breast cancer cells beyond the reach of surgery	Percent of operable patients bearing the numbers of tumour cells indicated					
	Negative nodes		1–4 positive nodes		>4 positive nodes	
	30d	40d	30d	40d	30d	40d
0	65	65	36	36	14	14
1 or <	80	74	56	47	22	17
10^1 or <	82	77	59	51	26	18
10^2 or <	85	80	63	56	30	22
10^3 or <	88	82	69	59	39	26
10^4 or <	90	86	73	65	45	33
10^5 or <	43	89	78	70	52	42
10^6 or <	95	93	83	78	63	53
10^7 or <	97	96	89	85	76	67
10^8 or <	99	99	94	92	88	85
10^9 or <	100	100	100	100	100	100

From Skipper (1975).

TABLE 7

Estimates of residual tumour burdens in amputated osteogenic sarcoma patients assuming overall doubling times of 10, 15 or 20 days for metastatic cells

Viable tumour cells beyond the reach of surgery	Percent of patients in which local control was achieved		
	10d	15d	20d
0	18	18	18
1 or <	32	21	19
10^1 or <	38	23	19
10^2 or <	42	25	20
10^3 or <	47	35	23
10^4 or <	59	39	27
10^5 or <	69	48	38
10^6 or <	76	65	48
10^7 or <	90	76	69
10^8 or <	97	95	90
10^9 or <	100	100	100

From Skipper (1975).

allowing the placement on a quantitative basis of discussions of therapeutic strategies. It seems evident in fact that different treatments as regards choice of agents (cell cycle-specific viz. non-specific) and the duration of treatment will be required for mammary cancer patients with 4 or more positive nodes at diagnosis in respect to individuals with negative or less than 4 involved nodes.

The obvious yardstick of concepts developed at the animal levels is their successful application in the clinic. It is thus more than rewarding that the above expounded rationale for initiation of chemotherapy of disseminated cells as soon as possible after non-curative intervention of the primary tumour with surgery (i.e. prophylactic chemotherapy of undetectable, micrometastases (Schabel, 1975b), has proven valid in man. The remarkable successes recently obtained with early post-surgical adjuvant chemotherapy in mammary cancer (Fisher *et al.*, 1975; Bonadonna *et al.*, 1976) and osteogenic sarcoma (Jaffe *et al.*, 1974; Cortes *et al.*, 1975) lead us to hope that the same philosophy will be applied without delay to other neoplastic conditions with high risk of metastatic spread at the time of clinical diagnosis.

III. The Problem of Model Systems

A consideration, however brief, of model systems appears necessary in any discussion of metastasis formation because of the intimate connection of this problem with the possibility to progress in the understanding of the basic biology of the process and, consequently, to develop more effective and/or alternative methods for interfering with it.

It is apparent that the establishment of a metastasis is the final result of a complex series of events in which an array of competing and synergistic factors, both intrinsic and extrinsic to the malignant cell, are interplaying. An analysis of this complex chain is presented elsewhere in this volume and Fig. 2 suffices to recall the main phases in which the process can be conceptually divided, whereas Table 8 shows a motley of factors currently known to influence one of the crucial events in metastatic spread. It is also unnecessary to emphasize that our current knowledge of the various mechanisms intervening at each of these levels is essentially restricted to the small emerging tip of the iceberg. Current possibilities for an "in depth" analysis of the different steps identified above are still limited and available experimental conditions, though not entirely non-existent, need a great deal of expansion.

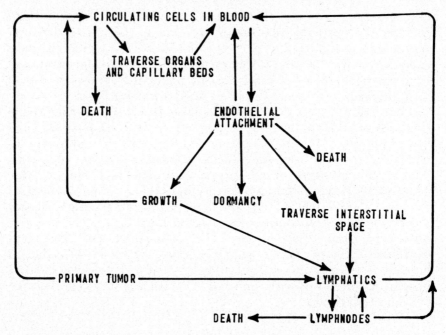

F$_{IG}$. 2. A schematic view of neoplastic dissemination (from Fisher and Fisher, 1967a)

Experimental systems of cancerous dissemination and metastasis formation can pragmatically be divided into complete models, such as those represented by the spontaneously metastatising animal neoplasms, and partial systems which aim to reconstruct only one or few of the steps in a whole complex. Spontaneous or induced rodent tumours which have been identified to reliably metastastise with consistent patterns, are not very common (Foulds, 1969), although their list appears to have been enlarging in the last few years. No attempts have been made to create an exhaustive catalogue and

T$_{ABLE}$ 8

A list of factors influencing the arrest of
tumour cell emboli in capillary beds

—embolic size and homogeneity
—tumour cell membrane charge
—tumour cell surface enzymes
—tumour cell plasticity
—host blood clotting mechanisms
—endothelial wall properties
—host immune mechanisms

mention will be restricted only to those tumours which have so far been the object of greater attention and/or with which we have had greater experience. In this category, the first place undoubtedly goes to the Lewis lung (3LL) tumour, a poorly differentiated epidermoid carcinoma that arose spontaneously in the lung of a C57Bl mouse in 1951 (Sugiura and Stock, 1955) and which when transplanted i.m. or s.c. gives visible metastases in the lungs of practically 100% of compatible hosts. As mentioned, this tumour has been analysed as regards its cytokinetic characteristics (Simpson-Herren et al., 1974), and is sensitive to a comparatively reasonable number of chemotherapeutic agents, cell kill being directly measurable by the procedures described by Steel and Adams (1975). In addition, since this tumour is antigenic, although feebly, it is also suitable for immunotherapeutic studies (Spreafico et al., 1975) and its growth has recently been shown to be accompanied by changes in various hematocoagulative parameters (Poggi et al., 1977) whose relevance and relationship with metastasis formation are however, still unresolved. Metastatic spreading of the 3LL tumour is rapid and surgery of the primary s.c. tumour 3 days after transplantation of 25 mg fragments is followed by only 85% cures (Skipper, 1974); surgery after day 10 does not result either in cures or in significant increase in survival time leading to the conclusion that by this time, additional cell dissemination from the primary does not contribute to the eventually lethal metastatic burden. With the inoculum usually employed in our Institute, i.e. $2 \cdot 10^5$ cells i.m., dissemination is somewhat less rapid: surgery at day 6 still gives 90% cures and amputation on day 10 gives no cures but still a significant increase in lifespan over non-amputated controls.

One important feature of the i.m. 3LL model is that, in non-amputated mice, death is not dependent on the extent of detectable lung involvement (see Table 9) but rather on the reaching by the primary of a lethal mass which, with most sub-lines, is in the 6–9 grams range. Also frequently employed for adjuvant chemotherapy studies, is the B16 melanoma; this tumour which arose spontaneously in a C57Bl mouse in 1954, grows s.c. only slightly less rapidly than the 3LL and it has been calculated to have a median overall cell doubling time from 1 cell to the lethal number, of $1 \cdot 4$ days versus $1 \cdot 2$ and $0 \cdot 5$ days for the 3LL and L1210 leukaemia respectively (Skipper, 1974). When transplanted in small solid 25–30 mg fragments it metastasises predominantly to the lungs and to other sites (kidney, brain, viscera) but less uniformly and rapidly than is seen with the 3LL tumour. In fact, surgical removal of the primary 6–8 days after standard inocula gives 40–50% cures; no cures are seen

TABLE 9

Effect of Triton WR 1339 on cancerous spreading by Lewis lung carcinoma in C57Bl/mice

Exp. group	Dose (mg/kg i.p.)	Schedule	Mean survival (days)	Primary tumour weight (g ± S.E.)	No. lung metast./ mouse
Control	—	—	31	6·1 ± 0·4	38 ± 3
TWR 1339	200	0–10	29	6·5 ± 0·3	15 ± 3*
TWR 1339	200	0–25	27	5·1 ± 0·6	10 ± 7*
TWR 1339	200	15–25	28	6·2 ± 0·5	14 ± 3*

* = $p < 0.05$. Tumour inoculum was of 2×10^5 cells i.m.

when surgery is applied at 15–18 days but significant increases in survival times are observable, i.e. the primary is still disseminating lethally effective cells. The B16 melanoma is poorly responsive to chemotherapy, since according to available data, even the best current drug combination does not kill more than 10^3–10^4 cells; however this tumour presents one of the clearest model conditions for evidence of the value of adjuvant chemotherapy and the importance of staging for an effective treatment.

Martin and his group (Martin et al., 1970; Stolfi et al., 1971; Anderson et al., 1974) have described a mammary adenocarcinoma originally induced by neonatal viral infection in (Balb/c × DBA/8)F$_1$ mice which metastasises with reasonable predictiveness. Visible lung metastases are found in approximately 80% of 10-month-old females of this strain and are observable with an incidence of 15% at 1–3 weeks after clinical detection of the primary, 25% at 4–6 weeks and 55% at 7–9 weeks, the extent of metastatic spread being related to the size of the primary rather than to the time required to reach this size. This tumour has also been characterized immunologically (Stolfi et al., 1974) and was one of the very first models in which the potential of surgery-chemotherapy was demonstrated. Corbett et al. (1975) have described a series of chemically induced colon carcinoma sub-lines with different metastatising capacities and for which the sensitivity to a series of cytotoxic agents has been tested, placing them in a category similar to B16 melanoma. Of interest, but needing further characterization, are the T241 fibrosarcoma of C57Bl/6 mice (Liotta et al., 1974) and line 1 alveolar carcinoma of Balb/c mice (Yuhas and Pazmiño, 1974) as the renal cell carcinoma described by Murphy and Hrushesky (1973). Various other metastatising neoplasms of mice and, less frequently, of rats, guinea-pigs and hamsters have also been employed by different groups for studies on selected aspects of the biology of tumour spreading and its inhibition (*see* for instance Gershon *et al.*, 1967, Griswold *et al.*, 1968; Ryan *et al.*, 1969; Zbar and Tanaka, 1971; Duff *et al.*, 1973; Karrer and Friedl, 1973; Bogden *et al.*, 1974; Currie and Alexander, 1974; Geddes-Dwyer *et al.*, 1974; Fisher *et al.*, 1974; Hagmar, 1974; Likhite and Halpern, 1974; Suurküla and Boeryd, 1974, and elsewhere in this volume). The conclusion is thus readily apparent that there is still need for a much more complete and interdisciplinarian characterization of many of these model tumours before their potential is properly assessed and exploited in cross-fertilization approaches. Lastly, one can hardly restrain from mentioning how the recent demonstration (Giovannella *et al.*, 1973; Helson *et al.*, 1975; Schmidt and Good, 1975) of metastasis formation by at least certain human tumours when transplanted in nude mice, opens a new and potentially rewarding avenue for investigating cancer spreading.

One of the most, if not the most, frequently employed condition for studying experimental metastasis has relied on the induction of lung nodules through the simple injection of dissociated tumour cells intravenously. Considering the complexity of the events leading to the eventual establishment and growth of a tumour secondary, there can be little doubt that this procedure is to be classified among the artificial partial models. The abruptness and transiency of the i.v. inoculum is obviously quite different from the more or less continuous dissemination of cells occurring in real conditions. More importantly, the presence of a primary sets in motion a whole array of changes in physiological parameters, for instance in the immune and coagulative status, which are obviously absent in the recipient of the injected cells. Reciprocal influences between the rates of growth of the metastasis and the primary malignancy have been described, although contrastingly, with various tumours in mice (Shatten, 1958; Ketcham *et al.*, 1961; Yuhas and Pazmiño, 1974). In addition, the cells injected are not necessarily those which would have spontaneously metastasised. This is equivalent to posing the question whether disseminated cells are simply a statistical cross-section of the entire tumour cell population, or whether the elements which after having settled into a new organ will eventually grow into a metastasis, possess different intrinsic properties from the rest of the disseminating and/or non-disseminating cells. Although preliminary indications favouring the second possibility have been presented by Fidler (1973 ; 1975) and more recently confirmed by us (Spreafico *et al.*, 1967a), the question is still unresolved. Model systems are just as useful as both their limits as well as potentials are clearly realized, therefore these caveats cannot obscure the value of this simple procedure for investigations of specific problems of metastatic spread and especially of approaches to its treatment.

A number of other *in vivo* or *in vitro* partial models of variable complexity have been described. Systems for the reconstruction of the first step in dissemination, i.e. tissue invasion, exist although they are far from satisfactory and the number of studies is still very limited. Two-dimensional monolayer systems (Abercrombie, 1967 ; Ambrose, 1967 ; Barski and Belehradek, 1968) in which tumour invasiveness is essentially evaluated by the capacity of the malignant cells to compress or migrate over the surface of normal elements, are difficult to interpret since some normal cells are also capable of moving under each other. In addition, the artificial substrates on which the migration occurs obviously play an un-physiological role. Three-dimensional *in vitro* or *in vivo* systems such as those described by Wolff (1967), Schleich (1973), Leighton (1968) or Easty and Easty (1974), although in principle a step closer to the real condition, are nevertheless still a long way from it, even in the light of our current very meagre understanding. Perfusion techniques for the study of the rate of tumour cell release have been described by several groups (Fisher and Fisher, 1967a ; Griffiths and Salsbury, 1965) ; among the most recent reports those of Butler and Gullino (1975) and Liotta *et al.* (1974) are especially informative on the high level of cell shedding which normally occurs with at least some tumours. We have also described (Spreafico and Garattini, 1974) a technically simple artificial condition which allows the semi-quantitative evaluation, through bioassay, of hematogenous dissemination after intracerebral implantation of tumour cells ; the system is essentially an expanding reservoir of malignant cells with a progressively increasing dissemination to the lungs and has been employed for the search of agents which could act on blood-borne neoplastic cells and/or at the level of organ entrapment. The latter phase can be quantitatively approached by the technique originally proposed by Fidler (1970) and by the use of isolated perfused organs (Guaitani *et al.*, 1973), a condition which has perhaps not been sufficiently explored in such types of studies. A reproducible condition for easily detectable lymphatic dissemination with macroscopic colonization of regional and extra-regional nodes is obtainable after tumour implants into the marrow cavity of long bones, such as the tibiae (Franchi *et al.*, 1968). A preferential or, at least temporarily, exclusive dissemination to the lymph nodes can be frequently obtained with intradermal or s.c. transplants of certain tumours (Carr and McGinty, 1974; Fisher *et al.*, 1974; Hanna and Peters, 1975; Kodama *et al.*, 1975) and Crile *et al.* (1971) have described a model in strain A mice where a syngeneic sarcoma transplanted in the foot progressively colonizes popliteal, iliac and tail nodes but secondaries in the viscera are seldom seen if the primary is left undisturbed despite the presence of cells in the circulation. A selective metastatic spread to lymph nodes and spleen is associated with certain reticulum cell sarcomas (Pilgrim, 1969; Parks, 1974), whereas liver metastasis, a condition of considerable clinical interest which is seldom seen as a predominant feature in metastasising complete systems in animals, can be obtained with relative ease after tumour implants in the coecum (Spreafico and Garattini, 1974). To the best of our knowledge, spontaneous bone metastases have been described only with murine plasmocytomas (Potter *et al.*, 1957).

The conclusion thus emerging from this admittedly sketchy review is somewhat mixed: although we are still wanting in economical, reproducible and sufficiently representative models for the analysis of various aspects of metastasis formation, at the same time it appears that a number of different conditions are already available which should allow the more in-depth investigations needed and which, moreover, have proven value for advancing clinically transposable therapeutical principles.

The conclusion (*see* below) that "alternative" anti-metastatic treatments exist and/or are foreseeable, appears to give a further dimension to the problem of model systems. Although present possibilities for such specific and selective interference with cancerous dissemination are still limited and whatever the ultimate clinical exploitability of such type of approaches will be, the question can be posed whether current screening procedures are suitable for revealing agents with such type of activity. This problem has been discussed (Spreafico and Garattini, 1974) and at the present time the answer is essentially negative and we regard it as an unfortunate limitation. In fact, although a number of test conditions *in vivo* and/or *in vitro* would in principle be necessary for revealing compounds acting on every possible level where interference with dissemination could be exerted, still it seems possible that through relatively minor changes in protocols and screening endpoints, significant advances in this direction could be made even employing experimental neoplasms already employed for screening purposes such as the 3LL tumour.

IV. Prospects for Alternative Anti-metastasis Treatment

The question that will be approached in this section is, simply stated, the following: is it possible to envisage pharmacological ways of interfering with cancer dissemination alternative to the use of "classical" chemotherapy and immunotherapy? Since metastasis formation is a characteristic restricted to neoplastic cells, agents which would be capable of specifically interfering with this process at any of its levels may, in principle, offer fruitful new possibilities to adjuvant cancer treatment which would, theoretically, have the advantage of selectivity. In this context, an ideal anti-metastatic agent would, in fact, act through mechanisms other than direct inhibition of the cell reproductive integrity, thus sidestepping the intrinsic limits of available cancer chemotherapeutic drugs and deriving from their non-specificity for malignant cells.

The search for agents possessing such an activity is still in its infancy and it seems fair to say that it has been often conducted more on pragmatic than on very rationalized bases in view of our substantial ignorance of many crucial events and/or mechanisms operative in cancer spread. The aim of presenting our past experience in this field is thus mainly to show that agents possessing such properties appear to exist and that beyond blocking the growth of established secondaries, there are in principle other levels at which interference with dissemination could be exerted. As an example of such "selective anti-metastatic" agents, Triton WR 1339, a polyoxyethylene ether of polymerized p-tertiary-octyl phenol-formaldehyde, could be mentioned. This non-ionic detergent is inactive in conventional screening employing a variety of experimental neoplasms amd is not cytotoxic *in vitro* even at high concentrations. However, treatment with this compound can markedly reduce the number of metastases in a variety (though not all) of experimental artificial or spontaneous conditions at doses without any inhibitory effect on the primary tumour growth (Tables 9 and 11). A more detailed discussion of the anti-disseminating activity *in vivo* of this prototype compound and of other polymers with similar effects has been presented (Franchi and Garattini, 1973; Ferruti *et al.*, 1973). In addition to a direct or indirect action on the transport and implantation phases of cancer spreading, and Triton WR1339 probably acts on these steps, other levels leading to metastasis formation may also offer possibilities for pharmacological interference. It is realized that as the division in steps of the entire process is an artifical conceptualization, also the classification of agents and/or approaches to restricted mechanisms is often a matter of semantics and is here used principally for exemplification purposes.

A first target may be represented by interference with the conditions in the tumour milieu which favour cell disaggregation and invasion of normal structures. It has been suggested that the invasiveness of malignant cells is due to their reduced adhesiveness (Zeidman, 1957; Humphreys, 1967) and local calcium deficiency was felt to be important (Humphreys, 1967); attempts to change serum calcium levels in the hope of influencing metastasis were without success, however (Fisher and Fisher, 1968). It has repeatedly been described (Gullino, 1973; Sylvèn, 1974) that the composition of the interstitial fluid in tumours is different from that of normal organs as regards, for instance, the concentration and/or activity of a series of lysosomal and cytoplasmic enzymes such as proteases and collagenolytic enzymes, which could attack the intercellular matrix and favour tumour invasiveness. Although the role played by such factors in neoplastic dissemination has not yet been sufficiently explored, if proven of pathogenic relevance means can be envisaged for influencing these changes in the tumour micro-environment. Recently, cells of B16 melanoma sub-lines selected for enhanced metastasising capacity *in vivo* have been found to possess elevated levels of proteases and glycosidases as compared to sub-lines of the same neoplasm with lower metastasising ability (Bosmann *et al.*, 1973). Protease inhibitors have been found to reduce the invasion of normal cell monolayers by malignant elements *in vitro* (Latner *et al.*, 1973). The existence of a tumour permeability and of a chemotactic factor for tumour cells have been described (Ozaki *et al.*, 1971; Koono *et al.*, 1974) as well as that of glue-like materials favouring cellular adhesion (Maslow and Weiss, 1972); it is clear that these factors could well be targets for interference or control.

Another target to which attention has already been drawn is represented by the attempt to a normalization of tumour vasculature; it is known that tumours possess angiogenic capacity which appears to be mediated by at least one distinct factor (Folkman, 1974) and the rudimental nature of the neovascularization at the periphery or within the primary tumour mass has been indicated as one important anatomical basis for neoplastic dissemination. Normalization of the tumour vasculature has been recognized as a distinguishing mechanism of ICRF 159 (Hellmann and Burrage, 1969; Salsbury *et al.*, 1974), the best known member of the bis-dioxopiperazine class of agents. This compound is capable of significantly reducing metastasis formation after treatments having no effect on the primary tumour (Table 10). The same table shows on the other hand, that the inhibition of metastases obtained with an agent such as Cyclophosphamide is proportional to the reduction in primary tumour weight. Although ICRF 159 possesses also a direct cytotoxic activity thus preventing its placement in the category of ideal anti-metastatic agents as defined above, this combined activity on cell reproduction, and on the vessels is an example of types of approaches to cancer treatment holding clear potential, especially considering that other agents (*see* Spreafico and Garattini, 1974) have been reported to inhibit neo-vascularization.

TABLE 10

Effect of ICRF 159 and Cyclophosphamide on Lewis lung carcinoma in C57B1/6 mice

Exp. group	Dose (mg/kg i.p.)	Primary tumour weight (g ± S.E.)	Lung metast. weight (mg)	% Mice with metast.
Control	—	5·5 ± 0·1	26·5 ± 3·1	100
ICRF 159	30	2·9 ± 1·1*	1·8 ± 0·6*	50
	15	4·9 ± 1·5	3·1 ± 1·2*	66
	7·5	7·6 ± 1·1	3·1 ± 2·0*	100
Cyclo-P	127	1·0 ± 0·3*	0·2 ± 0·1*	12
	65	4·4 ± 0·2*	5·3 ± 1·1*	83
	32	5·8 ± 0·3	9·1 ± 1·4*	100

* $= p < 0.5$. Animals were killed 25 days after the i.m. transplant of 2×10^5 tumour cells. ICRF 159 was given q3d on day 3–21; Cyclo-P was injected on days 3, 4 and 14, 15.

An additional level for possible selective interference with dissemination is represented by the cell membrane in the hope of rendering circulating elements more easily destroyable, less capable of implanting into normal organs or, in principle, of diverting them to more easily "curable" sites. Because of their capacity to bind to cell surfaces, various types of polyelectrolytes have been investigated for their possible effects on cancer dissemination (Hagmar, 1973; Moroson, 1973) but no clear conclusion as to their efficacy can yet be reached considering the contrasting results obtained, depending not only on the physico-chemical properties of the compound but also on the type of tumour and treatment employed. In addition it also seems possible that their mode of action is more complex than initially surmised, possibly also involving effects at the host level.

The possible importance of blood coagulation mechanisms in cancer dissemination has been the object of debate for many years

TABLE 11

Effect of surgery plus ICRF 159 or Triton WR 1339 on survival and metastatic dissemination of i.m. Lewis lung carcinoma in C57Bl/6 mice

Exp. group	Dose (mg/kg i.p.)	Schedule	Mean survival (days)	% Cures	No. lung metast. mouse
Surgery	—	—	33	0	27 ± 3
ICRF 159	30	q3d, 3–21	29	0	13 ± 5*
ICRF 159	120	q6d, 3–21	38*	20	6 ± 1*
Surgery + ICRF 159	30	q3d, 3–21	50*	40	14 ± 4
Surgery + ICRF 159	120	q6d, 3–21	62*	80	—
Surgery	—	—	30	0	25 ± 4
Surgery + TWR 1339	200	qd, 0–10	41*	20	21 ± 5
Surgery + TWR 1339	200	qd, 10–25	35	10	24 ± 3

* $= p < 0.05$.
Surgery was performed 10 days after the i.m. transplant of 2×10^5 tumour cells.

(Wood et al., 1961; Sträuli, 1966; Lee, 1968; Ketcham et al., 1971; Gastpar, 1972; Hoover and Ketcham, 1975) and a detailed analysis of the various direct and especially indirect evidence supporting this view is beyond the scope of this chapter. For instance, thrombocytopenia has been found to reduce metastases numbers and a direct relationship between the capacity of experimental tumours to induce platelet aggregation and their metastasising ability has been proposed (Gasic et al., 1968, Gasic et al., 1973). Microscopic studies of the entrapment phase have indicated that cancer cells adhere and penetrate the endothelium under the protection of a fibrin and platelet thrombus (Wood, 1971).* On the other hand, the fibrin network found at the invading periphery of many tumours has been suggested as important in supporting tumour growth (thrombin has also recently been shown to stimulate cell multiplication (Teng and Chen, 1975)) and as a lattice favouring cell containment as well as a shield against drug diffusion. Tumour cells have been found to possess procoagulant as well as fibrinolytic activities (Holyoke et al., 1972; Rifkin et al., 1974). This complex type of observation has

* At both the entrapment and invasion phases of dissemination, passive mechanisms probably act in conjunction with active characteristics of the cancer cells.

prompted a relatively large effort aimed at controlling dissemination through agents influencing the coagulative equilibrium. The outcome of treatments with heparin are contradictory and both decreased as well as increased incidences of metastases, especially beyond the lung filter, have been reported (Agostino and Cliffton, 1965; Fisher and Fisher, 1967b; Hagmar and Norrby, 1970; Hilgard et al., 1972). The initial reports (Wood et al., 1961; Fisher and Fisher, 1967b) of a significant anti-metastatic activity of Warfarin after i.v. injection of tumour cells have been extended also to spontaneously metastasising tumours (Hoover and Ketcham, 1975), an activity which could be blocked by concomitant treatment with vitamin K (Brown, 1973). Table 12 shows the effects of Warfarin at doses maintaining the coagulative capacity at 10–20% of normal, in mice bearing the 3LL tumour (Poggi et al., 1977). Fibrinolytic agents have been observed to decrease intravenous metastases (Agostino and Cliffton, 1963; Gastpar, 1972; Wood and Hilgard, 1973) but we, among others, could not confirm these findings in spontaneously disseminating systems (Donati and de Gaetano, unpublished results). Aspirin, a potent inhibitor of platelet aggregation, was reported as effective in preventing experimental metastasis from tumours capable of inducing in vitro platelet aggregation (Gasic et al.,

TABLE 12

Effect of Polymethacrylic acid and Warfarin treatments on metastatic dissemination of Lewis lung carcinoma in C57B1/6 mice

Agent	Schedule	Dose (mg/kg i.p.)	Primary tumour weight (g ± S.E.)		No. lung metast./mouse	
			Controls	Treated	Controls	Treated
Polymetha-crilic acid	qd 3–24	20	$6·9 \pm 0·6$	$4·3 \pm 0·4$*	23 ± 2	3 ± 1*
		10		$5·1 \pm 0·3$		8 ± 2*
		5		$5·8 \pm 0·5$		9 ± 3*
	q5d, 0–20	40	$6·3 \pm 0·4$	$6·5 \pm 0·4$	18 ± 3	9 ± 1*
	q5d, 0–20	40†		$7·0 \pm 0·5$		6 ± 1*
Warfarin	continuous, in drinking water	$7·5 \rightarrow 1·5$ (mg/l)	$7·3 \pm 0·4$	$6·7 \pm 0·4$	16 ± 2	9 ± 2*

* $= p < 0·05$.   † i.v. treatment.
Animals were injected with $2·10^5$ tumour cells i.m. and sacrificed 25 days after transplant.

1973) but again this finding has not always been confirmed (Kolenich *et al.*, 1972). In conclusion, the status of this problem is far from being settled in many important aspects, and a number of criticisms can be raised against many of the experimental conditions employed, such as the use of allogeneic tumour cell injections without constant control on the quality of the cell preparation infused (e.g. dissociated cells versus microemboli) or on the level of anticoagulation maintained. In addition, treatments have generally been conducted without taking into account the possible changes in hemostatic parameters induced by the tumour-bearing state nor, in the evaluation of effects, has it often been possible to exclude other biological activities exerted by the agents on the host or on the tumour cells. Heparin for instance, has been shown to reduce cell reproductive potential (Norrby, 1973) and induce lymphocytosis (Cronkite *et al.*, 1962). It would thus seem rash to employ such treatments in the clinic, as was advocated (Thornes, 1972; Elias *et al.*, 1973), until a much clearer picture at the experimental level has been obtained through a series of carefully controlled studies in a number of systems.

Although immunotherapy in metastasis treatment and/or prevention has been discussed elsewhere (*see Chapter VI*), one can hardly refrain from mentioning that its full potential has not yet been defined even at the animal level, whether employed singly or in combination with chemotherapy (especially within the frame of the "complementary" approach recently proposed (Spreafico *et al.*, 1976b). At least partially related to immunotherapy is the use of agents capable of mobilizing both malignant cells and normal blood elements, especially lymphocytes, from their deposits into the circulation (Ormai and de Clercq, 1969). Polymethacrylic acid possesses such an activity and has been shown to be effective in reducing metastasis (Table 12).

In conclusion, it appears that alternative, selective anti-metastatic treatment is no longer the object of pure speculation; although extensive investigation is necessary before the stage of a transfer to man of such type of approaches developed at the experimental level is reached, there already seems to exist the basis for looking at the future with a reasonable degree of optimism.

References

Abercrombie, M. (1967). *In* "Mechanisms of Invasion in Cancer" (P. Denoix, ed.), pp. 140–144. Springer-Verlag, Berlin.
Agostino, D. and Cliffton, E. E. (1963). *Ann. Surg.* **157**, 400–408.

Agostino, D. and Cliffton, E. E. (1965). *Ann. Surg.* **161**, 97–102.

Ambrose, E. J. (1967). *In* "Mechanisms of Invasion in Cancer" (P. Denoix, ed.), pp. 130–139. Springer-Verlag, Berlin.

Anderson, J. C., Fugmann, R. A., Stolfi, R. L. and Martin, D. S. (1974). *Cancer Res.* **34**, 1916–1920.

Barski, G. and Belehradek, J. Jr. (1968). *In* "The Proliferation and Spread of Neoplastic Cells", pp. 511–530. Williams & Wilkins, Baltimore.

Bogden, A. E., Esber, H. J., Taylor, D. J. and Gray, J. H. (1974). *Cancer Res.* **34**, 1627–1631.

Bonadonna, G., Brusamolino, E., Valagussa, P., Rossi, A., Brugnatelli, L., Brambilla, C., De Lena, M., Tancini, G., Bajetta, E., Musumeci, R. and Veronesi, U. (1976). *New Engl. J. Med.* **294**, 405–410.

Bosmann, H. B., Bieber, G. F., Brown, A. E., Case, K. R., Gersten, D. M., Kimmerer, T. W. and Lione, A. (1973). *Nature, Lond.* **246**, 487–489.

Brown, J. M. (1973). *Cancer Res.* **33**, 1217–1224.

Butler, T. P. and Gullino, P. M. (1975). *Cancer Res.* **35**, 512–516.

Carr, I. and McGinty, F. (1974). *J. Pathol.* **113**, 85–95.

Corbett, T. H., Griswold, D. P. Jr., Roberts, B. J., Peckham, J. C. and Schabel, F. M. Jr. (1975). *Cancer Res.* **35**, 2434–2439.

Cortes, E. P., Holland, J. F., Wang, J. J. and Glidewell, O. (1975). *Cancer Chemother. Rep.* **6**, pt. 3: 305–313.

Crile, G. Jr., Isbister, W. and Deodhar, S. D. (1971). *Cancer*, **28**, 657.

Cronkite, E. P., Jansen, C. R., Mather, G. L., Nielsen, N. O., Usenik, E. A., Adamik, E. R. and Sipe, C. R. (1962). *Blood*, **20**, 203–213.

Currie, G. A. and Alexander, P. (1974). *Br. J. Cancer*, **29**, 72–75.

DeWys, W. D. (1973). *J. Natl. Cancer Inst.* **50**, 783–789.

Donati, M. B. and de Gaetano, G. Unpublished results.

Donelli, M. G. and Spreafico, F. (1976). In preparation.

Duff, R., Doller, E. and Rapp, F. (1973). *Science*, **180**, 79–81.

Easty, D. M. and Easty, G. C. (1974). *Br. J. Cancer*, **29**, 36–49.

Elias, E. G., Sepulveda, F. and Mink, I. B. (1973). *J. Surg. Oncol.* **5**, 189–193.

Ferruti, P., Danusso, F., Franchi, G., Polentarutti, N. and Garattini, S. (1973). *J. Med. Chem.* **16**, 496–499.

Fidler, I. J. (1970). *J. Natl. Cancer Inst.* **45**, 773–782.

Fidler, I. J. (1973). *Nature, New Biol.* **242**, 148–149.

Fidler, I. J. (1975). *Cancer Res.* **35**, 218–224.

Fisher, B., Carbone, P., Economou, S. G., Frelick, R., Glass, A., Lerner, H., Redmond, C., Zelen, M., Band, P., Katrych, D. L., Wolmark, N. and Fisher, E. R. (1975). *New Engl. J. Med.* **292**, 117–122.

Fisher, B. and Fisher, E. R. (1967b). *Cancer Res.* **27**, 421–425.

Fisher, B. and Fisher, E. R. (1968). *Cancer Res.* **28**, 1753–1758.

Fisher, B., Saffer, E. and Fisher, E. R. (1974). *Cancer*, **33**, 631–636.

Fisher, E. R. and Fisher, B. (1967a). *In* "Methods in Cancer Research" (H. Busch, ed.), Vol. 1, p. 243. Academic Press, New York and London.

Folkman, J. (1974). *Cancer Res.* **34**, 2109–2113.

Foulds, L. (1969). *In* "Neoplastic Development", Vol. 1. Academic Press, New York and London.

Franchi, G. and Garattini, S. (1973). *In* "Chemotherapy of Cancer Dissemination and Metastasis" (S. Garattini and G. Franchi, eds.), pp. 293–305, Raven Press, New York.

Franchi, G., Reyers-Degli Innocenti, I., Rosso, R. and Garattini, S. (1968). *Int. J. Cancer* **3**, 765–770.

Frei, E. III (1972). *Cancer Res.* **32**, 2593–2607.

Gasic, G. J., Gasic, T. B., Galanti, N., Johnson, T. and Murphy, S. (1973). *Int. J. Cancer*, **11**, 704–718.

Gasic, G. J., Gasic, T. B. and Stewart, C. C. (1968). *Proc. Natl. Acad. Sci. USA*, **61**, 46–52.

Gastpar, H. (1972). *Haematol. Rev.* **3**, 1–51.

Geddes-Dwyer, V., Bosanquet, J. S., O'Grady, R. L. and Cameron, D. A. (1974). *Pathology*, **6**, 71–78.

Gershon, R. K., Carter, R. L. and Kondo, K. (1967). *Nature, Lond.* **213**, 674–676.

Giovannella, B. C., Yim, S. O., Morgan, A. C., Stehlin, J. S. and Williams, L. J. (1973). *J. Natl. Cancer Inst.* **50**, 1051–1053.

Griffiths, J. D. and Salsbury, A. J. (1965). *In* "Circulating Cancer Cells". C. C. Thomas, Chicago.

Griswold, D. P. Jr., Schabel, F. M, Jr., Wilcox, W. S., Simpson-Herren, L. and Skipper, H. F. (1968). *Cancer Chemother. Rep.* **52**, 345–387.

Griswold, D. P. Jr., Simpson-Herren, L. and Schabel, F. M. Jr. (1970). *Cancer Chemother. Rep.* **54**, 337–346.

Guaitani, A., Bartošek, I. and Garattini, S. (1973). *In* "Chemotherapy of Cancer Dissemination and Metastasis" (S. Garattini and G. Franchi, eds.), pp. 307–314. Raven Press, New York.

Gullino, P. M. (1973). *In* "Chemotherapy of Cancer Dissemination and Metastasis" (S. Garattini and G. Franchi, eds.), pp. 89–95. Raven Press, New York.

Hagmar, B. (1973). *In* "Chemotherapy of Cancer Dissemination and Metastasis" (S. Garattini and G. Franchi, eds.), pp. 261–268. Raven Press, New York.

Hagmar, B. (1974). *Acta Pathol. Microbiol. Scand. (Sect. A)*, **82**, 379–385.

Hagmar, B. and Norrby, K. (1970). *Int. J. Cancer*, **5**, 72–84.

Hanna, M. G. and Peters, L. C. (1975). *Cancer*, **36**, 1298–1304.

Hellmann, K. and Burrage, K. (1969). *Nature, Lond.* **224**, 273–275.

Helson, L., Das, S. K. and Hajdu, S. I. (1975). *Cancer Res.* **35**, 2594–2599.

Hilgard, P., Beyerle, L., Hohage, R., Hiemeyer, V. and Kübler, M. (1972). *Eur. J. Cancer*, **8**, 347–352.

Holyoke, E. D., Frank, A. L. and Weiss, L. (1972). *Int. J. Cancer*, **9**, 258–263.

Hoover, H. C. Jr. and Ketcham, A. S. (1975). *Cancer*, **35**, 5–14.

Humphreys, S. R. and Karrer, K. (1970). *Cancer Chemother. Rep.* **54**, 379–392.

Humphreys, T. (1967). *In* "The Specificity of Cell Surfaces" (B. Davis and L. Warren, eds.), p. 195. Prentice-Hall Inc., Englewood, N.J.

Hutchison, D. J. and Schmid, F. A. (1973). *In* "Drug Resistance and Selectivity" (E. Mihich, ed.), pp. 73–126. Academic Press, New York and London.

Jaffe, N., Frei, E. III., Traggis, D. and Bishop, Y. (1974). *New Engl. J. Med.* **291**, 994–997.

Karle, H., Ernst, P. and Killmann, S. A. (1973). *Br. J. Haematol.* **24**, 231–244.

Karrer, K. and Friedl, H. P. (1973). *In* "Chemotherapy of Cancer Dissemination and Metastasis" (S. Garattini and G. Franchi, eds.), pp. 361–365. Raven Press, New York.

Ketcham, A. S., Sugarbaker, E. V., Ryan, J. J. and Orme, S. K. (1971). *Am. J. Roentgenol. Radium Therapy Nucl. Med.* **111**, 42–47.

Ketcham, A. S., Wexler, H. and Mantel, N. (1961). *J. Natl. Cancer Inst.* **27**, 1311–1321.

Kodama, T., Gotohda, E., Takeichi, N., Kuzumaki, N. and Kobayashi, H. (1975). *Cancer Res.* **35**, 1628–1636.

Kolenich, J. J., Monsour, E. G. and Flynn, A. (1972). *Lancet,* **2**, 714.

Koono, M., Ushijima, K. and Hayashi, H. (1974). *Int. J. Cancer,* **13**, 105–115.

Latner, A. L., Longstaff, E. and Pradhan, K. (1973). *Br. J. Cancer,* **27**, 460–464.

Lee, Y. N. (1968). *Mod. Med.* **65**, 36–39; 123–128; 205–210.

Leighton, J. (1968). *In* "The Proliferation and Spread of Neoplastic Cells", pp. 533–551. Williams & Wilkins, Baltimore.

Likhite, V. V. and Halpern, B. N. (1974). *Cancer Res.* **34**, 341–344.

Liotta, L. A., Kleinerman, J. and Saidel, G. M. (1974). *Cancer Res.* **34**, 997–1004.

Martin, D. S., Hayworth, P. E. and Fugmann, R. A. (1970). *Cancer Res.* **30**, 709–716.

Maslow, D. E. and Weiss, L. (1972). *Exp. Cell Res.* **71**, 204–208.

Mayo, J. G., Laster, W. R. Jr., Andrews, C. M. and Schabel, F. M. Jr. (1972). *Cancer Chemother. Rep.* **56**, 183–195.

Moroson, H. (1973). *In* "Chemotherapy of Cancer Dissemination and Metastasis" (S. Garattini and G. Franchi, eds.), pp. 245–252. Raven Press, New York.

Murphy, G. P. and Hrushesky, W. J. (1973). *J. Natl. Cancer Inst.* **50**, 1013–1025.

Norrby, K. (1973). *In* "Chemotherapy of Cancer Dissemination and Metastasis" (S. Garattini and G. Franchi, eds.), pp. 269–277. Raven Press, New York.

Ormai, S. and De Clercq, E. (1969). *Science,* **163**, 471–472.

Ozaki, T., Yoshida, K., Ushijima, K. and Hayashi, H. (1971). *Int. J. Cancer,* **7**, 93–100.

Parks, R. C. (1974). *J. Natl. Cancer Inst.* **52**, 971–973.

Pilgrim, H. I. (1969). *Cancer Res.* **29**, 1200–1205.

Poggi, A., Polentarutti, N., Donati, M. B., de Gaetano, G. and Garattini, S. (1977). *Cancer Res.* **37**, 272–277.

Potter, M., Fahey, J. L. and Pilgrim, H. I. (1957). *Proc. Soc. Exp. Biol. Med.* **94**, 327–333.

Rifkin, D. B., Loeb, J. N., Moore, G. and Reich, E. (1974). *J. Exp. Med.* **139**, 1317–1328.

Ryan, J. J., Ketcham, A. S. and Wexler, H. (1969). *Cancer Res.* **29**, 2191–2194.

Salsbury, A. J., Burrage, K. and Hellmann, K. (1974). *Cancer Res.* **34**, 843–849.

Schabel, F. M. Jr. (1969a). *In* "Neoplasia in Childhood", pp. 61–78. Year Book Med. Publ., Chicago.

Schabel, F. M. Jr. (1969b). *Cancer Res.* **29**, 2384–2389.

Schabel, F. M. Jr. (1975a). *Cancer,* **35**, 15–24.

Schabel, F. M. Jr. (1975b). *Am. J. Roentgenol. Radium Therapy Nucl. Med.* In press.

Schleich, A. (1973). *In* "Chemotherapy of Cancer Dissemination and Metastasis" (S. Garattini and G. Franchi, eds.), pp. 51–58. Raven Press, New York.

Schmidt, M. and Good, R. A. (1975). *J. Natl. Cancer Inst.* **55**, 81–87.

Shatten, W. E. (1958). *Cancer,* **2**, 455–459.

Sheehy, P. F., Fried, J., Winn, R. and Clarkson, B. D. (1974). *Cancer,* **33**, 28–37.

Shipley, W. U., Stanley, J. A. and Steel, G. G. (1975). *Cancer Res.* **35**, 2488–2493.

Simpson-Herren, L., Sanford, A. H. and Holmquist, J. P. (1974). *Cell Tissue Kinet.* **7**, 349–361.

Skipper, H. E. (1974). "Booklet 11", Southern Research Inst., Birmingham, Alabama.

Skipper, H. E. (1975). "Booklet 7", Southern Research Inst., Birmingham, Alabama.

Spreafico, F., Anaclerio, A. and Moras, M. L. (1967a). In preparation.

Spreafico, F. and Garattini, S. (1974). *Cancer Treatment Rev.* **1**, 239–250.

Spreafico, F., Tagliabue, A. and Mantovani, A. (1976b). *Cancer Immun. Immunother.* In press.

Spreafico, F., Vecchi, A., Mantovani, A., Poggi, A., Franchi, G., Anaclerio, A. and Garattini, S. (1975). *Eur. J. Cancer*, **11**, 555–563.

Steel, G. G. and Adams, K. (1975). *Cancer Res.* **35**, 1530–1535.

Stolfi, R. L., Martin, D. S. and Fugmann, R. A. (1971). *Cancer Chemother. Rep.* **55**, 239–251.

Stolfi, R. L., Fugmann, R. A., Stolfi, L. M. and Martin, D. S. (1974). *Int. J. Cancer*, **13**, 389–403.

Sträuli, P. (1966). *Thromb. Diath. Haemorrh. Suppl. 20*, **147**+.

Sugiura, K. and Stock, C. C. (1955). *Cancer Res.* **15**, 38–51.

Suit, H. D. and Maeda, M. (1967). *J. Natl. Cancer Inst.* **39**, 639–652.

Suurküla, M. and Boeryd, B. (1974). *Int. J. Cancer*, **14**, 633–641.

Sylvén, B. (1974). *Schweiz. Med. Wochen.* **104**, 258–261.

Tannock, I. F. (1969). *Cancer Res.* **29**, 1527–1534.

Teng, N. N. H. and Chen, L. B. (1975). *Proc. Natl. Acad. Sci. USA*, **72**, 413–417.

Thornes, R. D. (1972). *J. Irish College Phys. Surg.* **2**, 41–42.

Valeriote, F. and van Putten, L. (1975). *Cancer Res.* **35**, 2619–2630.

Wilcox, W. S., Griswold, D. P., Laster, W. R. Jr., Schabel, F. M. Jr. and Skipper, H. E. (1965). *Cancer Chemother. Rep.* **47**, 27–39.

Wolff, E. (1967). *In* "Mechanisms of Invasion of Cancer" (P. Denoix, ed.), pp. 204–211. Springer-Verlag, Berlin.

Wood, S. (1971). *In* "Pathobiology Annual", pp. 550–568. Appleton Century-Crofts, New York.

Wood, S. Jr. and Hilgard, P. H. (1973). *Johns Hopkins Med. J.* **133**, 207–213.

Wood, S. and Holyoke, E. D. and Yardley, J. H. (1961). *Can. Cancer Conf.* **4**, 167–223.

Yankee, R. A., De Vita, V. T. and Perry, S. (1967). *Cancer Res.* **27**, 2381–2385.

Yuhas, J. M. and Pazmiño, N. H. (1974). *Cancer Res.* **34**, 2005–2010.

Zbar, B. and Tanaka, T. (1971). *Science*, **172**, 271–273.

Zeidman, I. (1957). *Cancer Res.* **17**, 157–162.

Chapter V

Therapy of Metastatis Disease: Canine and Feline Models

L. N. OWEN

Department of Veterinary Clinical Medicine, School of Veterinary Medicine, Cambridge, England

I. Introduction

Many tumours of the dog and cat have a pathological appearance and natural history very similar to their counterpart in man. A survey of spontaneous neoplasms in dogs and cats has been conducted in two Californian counties by Dorn *et al.* (1968a) who found that of all neoplasms 4842 were from dogs, 621 from cats and 184 from other domestic species. The estimated annual incidence rates for cancer of all sites were 381·2/1000,000 dogs and 155·8/100,000 cats. The rate in dogs exceeded the annual incidence rate for all types of cancer in human residents. In dogs 34% of all neoplasms were malignant whereas in the cat 72% were malignant.

In a study by Priester and Mantel (1971) the relative risk value (R) of neoplasia was 0·9 for the Beagle with the Boxer heading the list with a value of 4·0 and the Pomeranian and Chihuahua with low R values of 0·4.

II. Natural History and Pathology

The more important tumours which are either good models for neoplasia in man or valuable models for basic studies are: mammary tumours, osteosarcoma, melanoma, lymphosarcoma, mastocytoma, and the transmissible venereal tumour.

A. *Mammary Tumours: Dog*

Mammary tumours are the most common single group of neoplasms in the bitch and account for over one quarter of all tumours. Dorn *et al.* (1968b) found an incidence rate of 105/100,000 of the population, whereas the incidence rate in cats was only 12·8/100,000. Histologically malignant tumours account for about half the total but metastasis does not occur in all these cases.

There are normally ten mammary glands in the bitch with the inguinal glands having more tumours, perhaps because these glands are larger than the anterior glands. Mammary neoplasms in the bitch originate from the epithelial cells which line ducts or alveoli. They also arise from myoepithelial cells which lie adjacent to duct or alveolar epithelium or from interstitial connective tissue or fat. Mixed mammary tumours which are common in the bitch and which can be benign or malignant, are extremely rare in women. These tumours arise from at least two of the above cell types and a wide variety of histological appearances is seen.

A classification of the tumours and dysplasias of the mammary gland of the dog has been made by Hampe and Misdorp (1974). They classify epithelial tumours as "complex" when they consist of cells resembling both secretory and myoepithelial cells. This is of some importance, as these tumours are biologically less malignant than tumours of the simple type when one only of these types of cell occurs.

Malignant mammary tumours in the bitch (Fig. 1) spread by the lymphatic and haematogenous routes as they do in women. The prognosis following the surgical excision of canine mammary neoplasms has been established by Bostock (1975). In a study of 320 bitches from which mammary neoplasms had been excised, dogs were followed up until death or at least two years post-surgery. The median survival times of animals bearing histologically benign tumours was at least 114 weeks, while for dogs with carcinomas it was 70 weeks. Only 43% of dogs with carcinoma eventually died as a result of tumour, but a more accurate prognosis was possible by subdividing these tumours into their different morphological types.

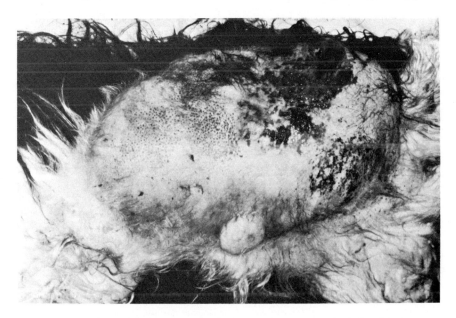

FIG. 1. Ulcerated, large mammary carcinoma of mammary glands in a bitch

Animals with solid or anaplastic carcinomas, had a significantly poorer survival time than those with papillary or tubular carcinomas and these particularly malignant tumours which metastasise widely are valuable models for breast carcinoma in women. The regional and distant lymph nodes are particularly involved in the metastatic process (Fig. 2) but frequently the lung, liver, kidney, spleen and other organs are also involved. Metastasis to bone producing both osteosclerotic and osteolytic lesions is recognized but is not found as frequently as in women. This may be because the disease process is

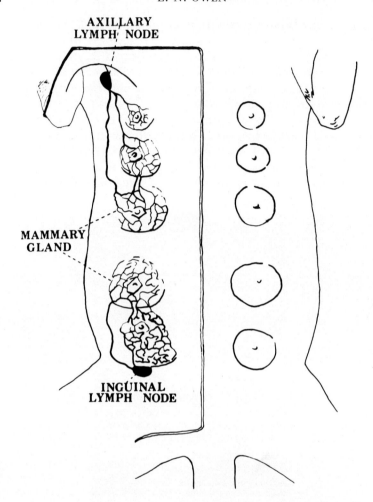

FIG. 2. The mammary glands in the bitch and their lymphatic drainage

not allowed to become complete in many instances as euthanasia is carried out on humane grounds. Moreover, very detailed skeletal studies are not usually performed. The role of vertebral venous spread is not known but this route of spread is anatomically possible.

B. *Mammary Tumours: Cat*

Unlike the dog the very large majority of feline mammary tumours are malignant (Fig. 3). Thus Hayden and Nielsen (1971) found 50 of

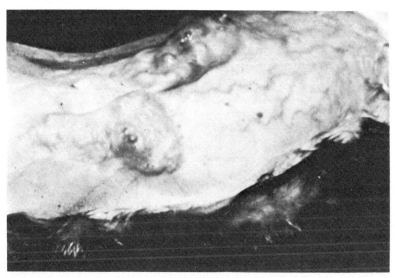

Fig. 3. Mammary carcinoma cat. Nearly all mammary tumours in the cat are carcinomas

55 tumours examined to be malignant. Twenty-seven were adeno-carcinomas, 19 papillary adenocarcinomas, 2 cirrhous and 2 anaplastic carcinomas.

An article by Weijer *et al.* (1972) has described the morphology and biology of 179 malignant mammary tumours in the cat and made some comparisons with canine and human mammary carcinomas. Unlike the dog, tumours were distributed evenly among the various glands in the cat. As in the dog, old animals were usually affected: the average age at first detection being 10·8 years. Following mastectomy survival times were usually only a few months.

Subdivision by histologic pattern showed 53 tubular adenocar-cinomas, 52 capillary adenocarcinomas, 35 solid carcinomas, 2 mucoid carcinomas, 34 compound tumours and 3 sarcomas. Histo-logic grading revealed that 50% of the low-grade malignancy group survived more than 1 year in contrast to 10% of the high-grade group.

Of the 129 necropsies made, 120 showed metastasis, most commonly in regional lymph nodes (82·8%), lungs (83·6%), pleurae (42·2%) and liver (23·6%).

C. *Osteosarcoma*

A comparative account of osteosarcoma in man and dog has been given by Owen (1969b). Most of the osteosarcomas in these species arise in the metaphysis of a long bone: common sites in the dog being the proximal humerus and distal radius in the weight-bearing forelimb (Fig. 4). Well over half the tumours in man occur in the distal femur and proximal tibia.

It is well known that osteosarcoma is mainly a disease of large dogs with the Wolfhound and Great Dane particularly being affected. An

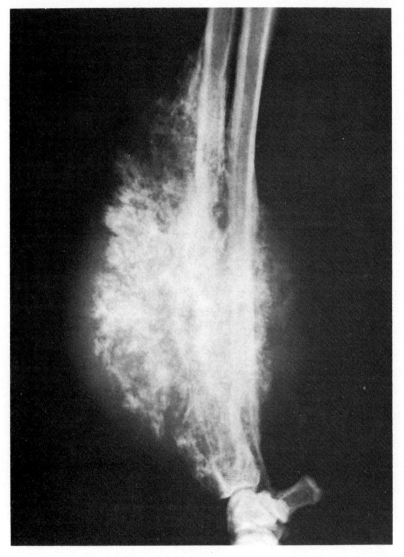

FIG. 4. Very advanced osteosclerotic osteosarcoma distal radius and ulna—Great Dane

association between tall stature and osteosarcoma in childhood has also been established (Fraumeni, 1967). Half of the cases in dogs occur between 5 and 9 years but in man the maximum mortality from limb-bone tumours occurs between 15 and 19 years, which is at a relatively younger age and in groups where the epiphyses have not fused. Both in man and dog, osteosarcoma metastasises early to the lungs with radiographic appearance of metastases usually occurring in the dog within a few weeks of diagnosis (Fig. 5) whereas in man there is usually a time-interval of several months after the initial diagnosis. Metastasis to bone occurs in about 25% of the cases in man but appears to be less common in the dog.

The radiographical and pathological appearance is very similar in the two species and the prognosis is equally poor. The tumour appears to be as radio-resistant in the dog as it is in man.

Because cures following amputation in the dog are almost unknown and because of its great similarity to the tumour in man, new methods of therapy are particularly worthwhile in this tumour. The tumour is not common but sufficient cases can be obtained at a few centres to run clinical trials. There are insufficient cases seen in the cat to be of real value as a model.

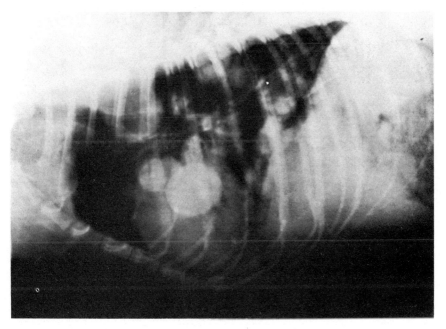

FIG. 5. Lung metastases in osteosarcoma—Wolfhound

D. *Melanoma: Dog*

Canine melanoma differs somewhat from that in man with regard to site distribution: in the dog the most malignant tumours are seen in the buccal cavity (Fig. 6) with frequent regional lymph node metastasis at the time of presentation. These tumours metastasise later to the lungs and sometimes to many other organs, including spleen, liver, kidney, central nervous system, pancreas, adrenal, heart and pituitary. Oral melanomas of man are rare and this difference probably reflects the greater degree of pigmentation in the mouths of dogs particularly affected, e.g. Cocker Spaniel, Scottish Terrier and Airedale. The cutaneous melanomas of the dog tend to be less malignant; only about 50% being progressive. These malignant cutaneous melanomas arise at a junctional naevus, tend to be locally invasive and show lymphatic migration to the regional lymph nodes and other organs.

Surgery is frequently successful in cases of benign cutaneous melanoma and malignant tumours of the skin can often be excised successfully in the early stages. In many other cases local or widespread metastases follow surgery. Oral melanomas involving the gum or hard palate can invade bone and render surgical removal difficult or impossible. Even in those cases where surgery seems feasible metastasis to regional lymph nodes, lungs or other sites is the usual end result.

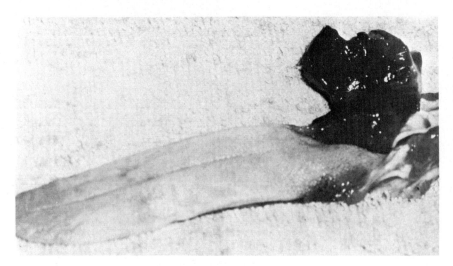

FIG. 6. Metastatic melanoma of buccal mucous membrane in tonsil—dog. This tumour metastasised widely

Some spontaneous melanomas in the dog are radiosensitive and one-year survival times can be obtained in some instances.

E. *Lymphosarcoma: Dog*

Lymphosarcoma in the dog is common and it is not difficult for a Veterinary School which is interested in this condition to deal with 50 cases a year. In the alimentary type of lymphosarcoma the small intestine is most often involved, the local lesion appearing as a firm annular thickening of the intestinal wall which has been infiltrated by a greyish-white homogenous tumour. The mesenteric lymph nodes are always involved and often many other organs also. Clinical signs in this type include anorexia and vomiting, diarrhoea or dysentery and as the prognosis is extremely poor, euthanasia is performed soon after a diagnosis is made. The prognosis in the thymic type is also very poor and treatment is seldom attempted.

In the more common, multicentric type there is usually bilateral symmetrical enlargement of the peripheral lymph nodes (Fig. 7) and tonsils with hepatosplenomegaly. The kidneys, lungs and other organs may sometimes be involved and some cases show an

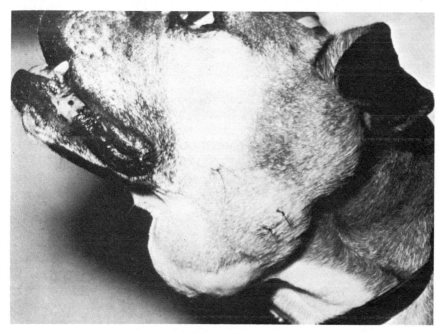

Fɪɢ. 7. Boxer showing greatly enlarged submandibular lymph node due to lymphosarcoma

infiltration of lymphocytes into the anterior chamber of the eye. Anaemia is usually present, probably due to depressed erythropoiesis and increased haemolysis. The white cell count is frequently raised due to a neutrophilia but in some cases there is an increase in lymphocytes or lymphoblasts. In more rare cases a true lymphocytic leukemia with a total w.b.c. count of 500,000 or more occurs. The dogs are usually very thin in these cases and have a marked hepatosplenomegaly but are often without marked peripheral lymph node enlargement.

Affected lymph nodes show a complete loss of normal architecture. The cortex and medulla are replaced by a homogenous sheet of lymphoid cells which contain large and small lymphocytes and lymphoblasts. Vacuolated histiocytes occur in some tumours leading to the so-called "starry-sky" appearance.

Most cases of multicentric disease in the dog are dead within 3 months of the first veterinary consultation.

F. *Lymphosarcoma: Cat*

Lymphosarcoma is the most common neoplasm in cats. The alimentary and thymic types are more common, the multicentric type occurring less frequently. Kidney involvement is also frequently seen in the cat and leads to progressive renal failure while liver involvement, particularly in old cats, is also common. Leukemia is uncommon but lymphocytic, myeloid and monocytic types can occur.

The disease in the cat is caused by an oncornavirus and is horizontally transmissible. In clinically affected cats, or in carriers, smears of peripheral blood or bone marrow treated with fluorescein-conjugated rabbit anti-feline leukemia virus serum show a light green fluorescence characteristic for the presence of virus. C-type particles are commonly seen on EM examination of many tissues (Fig. 8). The prognosis is very poor.

G. *Mastocytoma: Dog*

Mastocytomas, which account for about 10% of all skin tumours in the dog, are rare in man. These malignant tumours appear in sufficient numbers in dogs however, to make therapeutic studies worthwhile. There is a marked breed incidence, with Boxers and Boston Terriers being the most frequently affected. There is no predilection for any particular site in the skin and the tumours can be

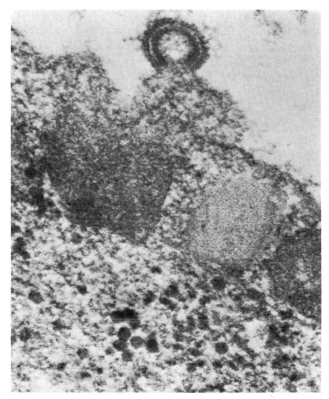

FIG. 8. Budding C-type particle—lymphosarcoma cat

single or multiple and either slow or fast growing. The rapidly growing tumours frequently invade and cause ulceration.

The tumours consist of a diffuse infiltration of dermal connective tissue by mast cells among which eosinophils are frequently found. Bostock (1973) has graded the tumours histologically and showed this to be of prognostic significance. The surgical removal of well-differentiated mastocytomas results in an 80% cure rate, whereas over 70% animals with poorly-differentiated tumours are subjected to euthanasia because of re-growth or metastasis. The mean survival time of this latter group post-operatively is on average only 18 weeks. Early metastasis is to the regional lymph nodes with advanced tumours being widely disseminated.

H. *Transmissible Venereal Tumour*

This tumour has no human counterpart but it is useful in

immunological studies concerned with transplantation and cancer. It is widely distributed throughout the world, occurring particularly in subtropical and tropical areas. The tumour is normally transmitted at coitus by whole cells and under natural conditions lesions are usually confined to the mucous membranes of the penis (Fig. 9) and vagina but can also occur in the mouth. The tumour whether growing on the penis, prepuce or vaginal vulval mucous membrane, usually appears as a pinkish friable mass with an ulcerated and infected surface. Under laboratory conditions cell suspensions can be made and when injected subcutaneously into outbred dogs, tumours will develop in most instances. Following injection at several sites, multiple tumours can be grown in one animal. Histologically the tumour is an undifferentiated round cell neoplasm with some cases having small clumps of cells surrounded by fine reticulin. In spite of its name the tumour is transplantable rather than transmissible and no evidence of viral aetiology has been found.

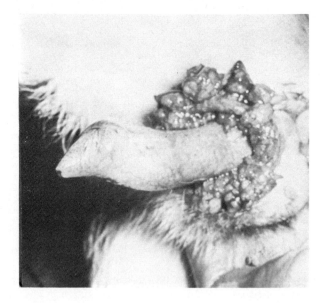

Fig. 9. Transmissible venereal tumour penis and prepuce of dog—Nigeria

Tumours from animals in widely different parts of the world have revealed a karyotype of 59 ± 5 instead of the normal 78 chromosomes.

Complete surgical removal is often difficult but the tumour is very radiosensitive. In some animals widespread metastasis occurs.

I. *Growth and Cell-population Kinetics of Spontaneous Tumours*

The relationship between cell proliferation and overall tumour growth rate is often difficult to obtain in human cancer. Owen and Steel (1969) measured visible metastases on serial radiographs in dogs and cats with various malignant tumours and obtained tumour volume doubling times of 7 to 150 days. Many tumours had doubling times between 20 and 40 days. The distribution of volume doubling times in these 9 animals when compared with the doubling times in a large number of tumours in men, is shown in Fig. 10. It will be seen that the doubling times in dogs are, on average, slightly shorter than the values for human tumours. They are, however, much longer than the doubling times seen in most rodent tumours. Tritiated thymidine was injected intravenously into these animals with measured tumours 1–2 hours before euthanasia and autoradiographic studies made. Calculation of the rate of cell production based on the measured thymidine labelling indices, were then usually found to be much higher than was necessary to maintain the observed growth rate and these results implied that extensive cell loss was taking place.

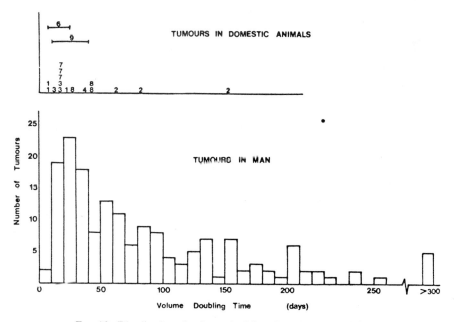

FIG. 10. Distribution of volume doubling times in man and dog

This cell loss factor, which is also well-recognized in human tumours, varied from 0–96%.

The cell population kinetics of the transmissible venereal tumour have been studied at two different stages of tumour growth using the labelled mitosis technique. At the first stage, the tumours were growing with a doubling time of about 4 days: at the second stage their growth rate was limited, probably by an immune reaction on the part of the host, to a doubling time greater than 20 days. The timing of the cell cycle was found to be similar in the rapidly growing tumours and in those growing more slowly. It was concluded that the slowing of growth was due to a considerable increase in the rate of cell loss as a result of the immune reaction (Cohen and Steel, 1972).

J. Transplantation and Tissue Culture Studies

While many of the spontaneous tumours are good models for therapy, they are not always available for such studies in sufficient numbers at the right time. Some results of value to a specific problem can be obtained using transplanted tumours which can be produced in large numbers.

Following the injection of 10^7–10^8 tumour cells into newborn dogs immunosuppressed with anti-canine lymphocyte serum, tumours usually grow within 2 to 6 months (Fig. 11). If malignant cells are injected intrafoetally at the 6th or 7th week of pregnancy, tumour growth in these dogs is usually visible between 2 to 6 months of birth. Tumours which have been successfully transplanted in this way include lymphosarcoma (Owen and Nielsen, 1968), lymphatic leukemia (Owen, 1971), osteosarcoma (Owen, 1969a), melanoma (Betton, 1975), fibrosarcoma (Owen, 1972) and mammary carcinoma (Owen and Morgan, 1975). The usual route of transplantation has been subcutaneous or intraperitoneal but tumour cells have also been injected intravenously (Fig. 12) and intra-arterially (Fig. 13). The histological appearance of the transplanted tumours is very similar to the original tumour but the doubling times are usually faster.

Cell lines of canine melanoma, osteosarcoma and solid mammary carcinoma have been established and proof of malignancy obtained by transplantation studies. While these transplanted tumours can be grown relatively quickly, they suffer from the disadvantage of all transplanted tumours in cancer research and since no syngeneic dogs are available, an additional disadvantage is that either a state of

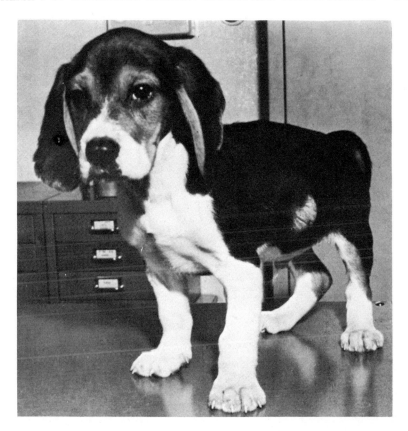

FIG. 11. Transplanted subcutaneous osteosarcoma growing in 2-month-old immunosuppressed Beagle

tolerance exists (intrafoetal injection) or the immune mechanisms are
suppressed by the antilymphocyte serum.

The transmissible venereal tumour can usually be transplanted
without previous immunosuppression of the recipient and mast cell
leukemia of the dog has been transmitted using cell-free filtrates
(Lombard *et al.*, 1963; Post *et al.*, 1969). Lymphosarcoma in the cat
occurs following the injection of FeLV virus, but in a high percentage
of cats other conditions, e.g. myeloid leukemia, atrophy of the
thymus, etc. are produced (Mackey *et al.*, 1972). Fibrosarcoma in the
cat is also virus transmitted (Snyder and Theilin, 1969). When this
virus is injected into neonatal dogs, tumours with the histological
appearance of fibrosarcomas are produced but these tumours usually
regress.

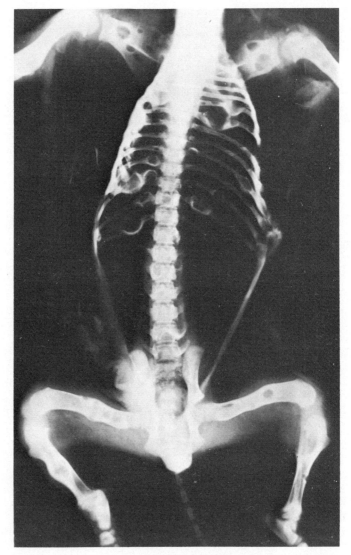

FIG. 12. Widespread transplanted osteosarcoma in bones following intravenous injection of cells grown in tissue culture

III. Radiotherapy

A. *Clinical Observations*

The response of tumours to radiotherapy is not so well-known in the

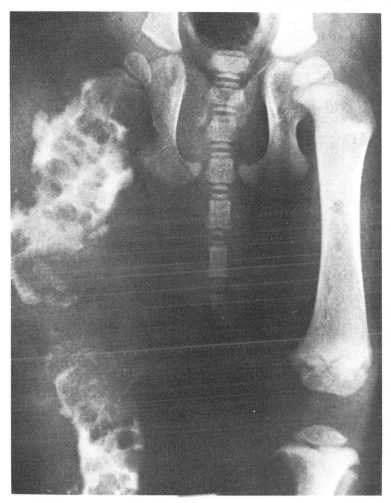

FIG. 13. Osteosarcoma of limb bones following injection of tumour cells into the external iliac artery

dog as in man. Most workers are agreed, however, that among the most radiosensitive tumours are the transmissible venereal tumour and the hepatoid tumours of the perianal region. Melanomas appear to respond better in the dog than in man (Silver, 1972) but cures are not often obtained because of metastatic spread. Squamous cell carcinomas have been reported to have a one year survival rate of 78% following radiotherapy (Silver, 1972) but X-irradiation of osteosarcomas using a Linear Accelerator (4500–5000 R) has only given survival times of 1 month to 1 year with an average of 4 months (Owen and Bostock, 1973).

The effects of single doses of X-irradiation on lung metastases in animals has been studied by van Peperzeel (1972). The doubling times of metastases in the lungs in 10 dogs were found to be between 8 and 31 days and in 2 of these dogs volume reduction curves following single doses of radiation to the metastatic tumour were determined. As previously recorded in man, a correlation was found between growth rate and radiosensitivity as judged from the volume reduction of the metastases. This was not dependent upon any particular histological appearance of the tumour. A period of accelerated growth was observed following this volume reduction. This period of accelerated growth, which also occurs following X-irradiation of tumours in mice and in humans, is important in so far as there could be a greater radiosensitivity during this period with second and third doses having a greater effect upon the volume reduction than the first dose of irradiation. Continuing research of this kind is yielding valuable information on X-irradiation of metastases.

The four factors known to affect fractionated radiotherapy are repair, repopulation, redistribution (of phases of differing sensitivity) and reoxygenation. In human patients it is likely that for most of the tumours treated by radiotherapy, the scheme with daily fractions used in most radiotherapy centres is close to the most effective one. However, it is possible that for rapidly-growing or slowly-growing tumours other and less regular fractionation schemes could give better results. In domestic animals studies on fractionation have been limited because of the necessity in most instances to anaesthetize the animal. Many of the animals are old and not good anaesthetic risks, so there has been a tendency to give bigger doses at larger intervals. Some well-conducted clinical trials on fractionation, however, would be of comparative interest.

Some of the primary and metastatic tumours appearing in domestic animals could also be used in trials of radiosensitizers. The most useful compounds at the moment appear to be those which mimic the electron-affinity property of oxygen but which are capable of diffusing further from capillary vessels because they are not rapidly metabolized in the cells. Toxicity tests of the nitro-imidazoles in experimental and tumour-bearing dogs are planned.

B. *Whole Body Irradiation*

A considerable amount of knowledge is available on the effects of whole body irradiation in dogs because of the attempts made to transplant various organs and bone marrow. Whole body X-irradiation has been tried therapeutically in lymphosarcoma but results were poor and it is unlikely to be any more successful, unless it is performed in laboratories fully equipped for the tissue typing of dogs. Studies on the biological behaviour of the transmissible venereal tumour when transplanted to dogs immunosuppressed with whole body X-irradiation have shown that the tumour adopts a regular malignant biological behaviour with widespread metastases (Cohen, 1973).

Observations on the effects of X-irradiation of an extra-corporeal circulation can readily be made in the dog because of its relatively large size.

A few studies on depression of circulating lymphocytes and the depression of the immune response following conventional radio-therapy for tumours in dogs have been conducted, but no figures are yet available which can be compared to those which have been published on women receiving radiotherapy for carcinoma of the breast (Stjernswärd, 1974): *see Chapter III*).

C. *Effect of "Prophylactic" X-irradiation of the Lung*

The poor prognosis following amputation of the affected limb in children with osteosarcoma has encouraged the development of radiotherapeutic or chemotherapeutic methods designed to kill as many tumour cells as possible in the lungs before they become radiographically visible. One series, where children received a total fractionated dose of 2000 R "prophylactically" to both lungs, showed that one- and two-year survival rates appeared to be improved but the 5-year survival rates were not obviously better than in children not X-irradiated (Newton, 1974). A further trial conducted by the European Organization for Research in the Treatment of Cancer is still in progress.

The same poor prognosis exists in the dog with metastases usually appearing, however, at a shorter time interval than occurs in man. Some trials have been made in the dog on the effects of X-irradiation of one lung (Owen and Bostock, 1973).

Following the intravenous injection of canine osteosarcoma cells in puppies immunosuppressed with anti-lymphocyte serum, one lung was fractionally X-irradiated to a total dosage of 600–1800 R. When these animals were examined at *post mortem* 2 5 weeks later, considerably less tumour was found on the X-irradiated side compared with the non-irradiated side. One lung was also pro-phylactically X-irradiated (2 × 600 R) in two dogs with spontaneous primary melanoma in which the primary tumour had been ablated. In these dogs, also, less tumour grew on the X-irradiated site (Fig. 14).

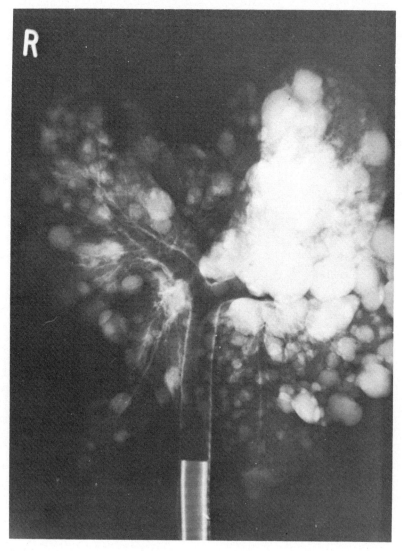

FIG. 14. Prophylactic X-irradiation of one lung for canine melanoma. Less tumour grew on the X-irradiation (R) side but this did not occur with osteosarcomas

In two other dogs with spontaneous osteosarcoma and two with carcinoma where the primary tumour was not completely destroyed, thoracic X-irradiation of one side resulted in more tumour developing in the X-irradiated lung than in the non-irradiated lung. The most dramatic result occurred in a dog with a metastasising tonsillar carcinoma where 56 macroscopic and multiple microscopic metastases occurred in the irradiated lungs, but none was found on the normal side. The results leave no doubt that X-irradiation was harmful in these four cases.

Although the number of clinical cases treated was small and the fractionation of radiation doses could be improved, two main conclusions can be drawn from this study: where the primary tumour is completely excised or otherwise killed, prophylactic X-irradiation of the lungs can delay the growth of a radiosensitive tumour. When the primary tumour is not completely excised or otherwise killed, prophylactic X-irradiation of the lung can sometimes increase the numbers of metastases. The exact mechanism of the X-irradiation effect is not known; damage to endothelium of blood vessels, depression of local immune response or the liberation of growth-stimulating substances are possibilities. Recent research in the dog in which one lung was X-irradiated and osteosarcoma cells labelled with Cr^{51} injected intravenously, has shown that the same number of tumour cells lodge in the X-irradiated side as on the non-irradiated side, i.e. the mechanism is not solely due to a "trapping" effect.

IV. Chemotherapy

A. *Drug Trials*

Drug resistance and toxicity remain two of the major problems in the treatment of tumours in the dog and cat as they are in humans. In the centre of large tumours drug penetration is also reduced due to the poor blood supply.

A quantitative comparison of toxicity of anti-cancer agents made in the mouse, rat, hamster, dog, monkey and man (Freireich *et al.*, 1966) has shown that on a mg/Kg basis the maximum tolerated dose (MTD) in man is about one-twelfth the LD_{10} in mice, one-tenth the LD_{10} in hamsters and one-seventh the LD_{10} in rats. The MTD in monkeys is about one-third that of man and in dogs it is about one-half the MTD in man. However, on a mg/M^2 basis, the MTD in man is about the same as each of these species. Due to the enormous differences in size between the toy breeds (e.g. Chihuahua) and the giant breeds (e.g. Great Dane) it is becoming more common in veterinary hospitals to prescribe cancer chemotherapeutic compounds in a mg/M² basis.

Equipped with the manufacturer's toxicity data on healthy dogs dosed with new chemotherapeutic drugs, caution is still required in the clinical application in tumour-bearing dogs and cats. As well as the more usual sites of toxicity such as the bone marrow (Fig. 15) and intestine, toxic effects on the kidney, particularly with alkylating agents, are common. Unlike the healthy young Beagles used in the pharmaceutical industry, clinical and subclinical nephritis is a common condition in dogs and cats of tumour-bearing age and additional insults can be fatal.

There are very few reports of chemotherapy for tumours in the cat. For lymphosarcoma, prednisone and vincristine or prednisone and cyclophosphamide have been given in 15 cats. All were, however, dead within 3 months of the onset of therapy (Squire and Bush, 1973). In general, cats with lymphosarcoma or advanced metastatic solid tumours do not make such good patients as dogs. Oral administration of drugs is frequently more difficult and refusal to eat in hospital accommodation is often encountered.

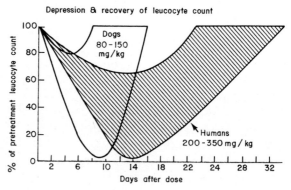

FIG. 15. Depression and recovery of leucocyte counts in dog and man following the intravenous injection of a tumour inhibiting epoxide (ethoglucid)

In the dog most reports have dealt with the treatment of multicentric lymphosarcoma using one of the alkylating agents, antifolinic acid compounds, and vinca alkaloids, L-asparaginase or the cortico-steroids. At some Veterinary Schools dogs with this tumour are available in sufficient numbers so that a trial on a new drug can be conducted. The currently best available therapy which produces objective regression (often dramatic) and approximate doubling of life expectancy without toxicity is a combination of vincristine, cytosine arabinoside, cyclophosphamide and prednisone (Bostock *et al.*, 1975). If regression is not complete by one month, L-asparaginase can be used in addition but care should be taken as anaphylaxis has occurred in some dogs given this drug. The limiting factor for many dog owners is the high cost of some of the drugs.

Squire and Bush (1973) have classified the lymphosarcomas in dogs seen by them into lymphocytic, undifferentiated and histiocytic types. They found their histiocytic tumours very resistant to prednisone therapy alone, but responding well to a mixture of prednisone, vincristine and cyclophosphamide.

Studies on chemotherapy in osteosarcoma have been made in which the alkylating agent ethoglucid (triethylene glycol diglycidyl ether) was used intra-arterially or by limb perfusion (Owen, 1962, 1964). The technique of limb perfusion using cross-matched blood and canulating the brachial or femoral vessels is a surgical technique not difficult in the large breeds of dogs which develop bone tumours. Despite concentrations of the drug in the limb which reached about 6 times the concentration which could be given systemically per weight of tissue, regressions were obtained for more than 2 months in only 5 of 15 dogs and the longest period of regression was only 5 months.

When canine osteosarcoma cells were cultured *in vitro* with 17 different drugs, the most marked cytopathic effects were shown by actinomycin D, vinblastine, vincristine, mycophenolic acid, and ethoglucid (Owen, 1973). If the vinca alkaloids are classified as one drug, it is interesting to note that the four compounds all have different cytotoxic actions.

Attempts at chemotherapy for canine metastatic bone tumours in the lungs when still of microscopic size have not yet been made. Trials of methotrexate and doxorubicin (adriamycin) similar to those in progress in the Medical Research Council Trial in man, could yield interesting comparative results. The time from amputation to death averages about 14 weeks in the dog so that results of new methods of therapy in the dog are obtained more quickly than those in man. A major problem is the limited number of dogs with osteosarcoma available at any one centre for such a study and the very few centres equipped or having the personnel with the interest to do such studies. Such centres are very few in the U.S.A., and in Great Britain at the present time only one centre is seriously interested in this problem. It is expected that some progress will be made by collaboration between centres, the work being coordinated by the therapy branch of the comparative oncology section of W.H.O.

Very few trials on sufficient numbers of animals have been made in dogs suffering from the other common solid malignant tumours. Remarkably good regressions have, however, been reported in mastocytomas, squamous cell carcinomas and mammary gland adenocarcinomas using mitogillin, a polypeptide produced by *Aspergillus restrictus* (NSC 69529) (Roga *et al.*, 1971). The very high success rate warrants confirmation as no further reports appear to have been made since 1971.

V. Hormonal Effects

A. *Mammary Gland*

In entire female cats approximately a seven-fold higher relative risk of mammary cancer exists than in ovariectomized cats. Therapeutic ovariectomy has been found, however, to be of little value in the few cases recorded.

Bitches ovariectomized before any oestrous cycle had approximately 0·5% of the mammary cancer risk, those with one oestrous cycle had 8% and animals that had 2 or more oestrous cycles before neutering had 26%. Within the group having 2 or more oestrous cycles, ovariectomy before 2·5 years of age was shown to produce a marked sparing effect on mammary cancer risk not shown in bitches neutered after 2·5 years of age. Ovariectomy after cancer diagnosis does not appear to affect the survival or cause of death (Schneider *et al.*, 1969). The long-held view of the value of ovariectomy in breast cancer in women has also been questioned (Ravdin *et al.*, 1970).

In the bitch the myo-epithelial component of the mammary gland is very important and it is perhaps here, in comparison with other species, that hormonal differences may lie. The roles of prolactin and growth hormone in the development of mammary tissue in the bitch are not clear at the present time. It is likely that progesterone stimulation increases the activity of the anterior pituitary gland. In Beagle bitches dosed over a long period of time with the potent progestogen and contraceptive drug, chlormadinone acetate, an acromegalic-like appearance and diabetes developed in the dogs (Hill and Dumas, 1973).

Growth of the mammary gland in the ovariectomized bitch follows the administration of progesterone alone, whereas in most species this requires the interaction of oestrogen. The mammary gland in the intact bitch readily produces fibroadenomatous and other pathological changes, including neoplasia in some instances, following the administration of progesterone or progestogens structurally related to the natural hormone. Progestogens structurally related to testosterone have not induced such effects in the dog (Hill and Dumas, 1973). The fibroadenomatous and other changes seen do not occur in other species treated similarly, with the possible exception of the ferret. In the dog the pharmacokinetic patterns of administered oestradiol differ considerably from those seen in man. The dog is primarily a faecal excretor of the steroid, whereas the major route in humans is urinary.

For these various reasons it is clear that the dog mammary gland is not an ideal model for studying hormones which are used as contraceptives in women. On somewhat less evidence it appears unlikely that hormonal studies on mammary cancer in dogs will prove as profitable to the human breast cancer problem as other studies, e.g. chemotherapy or immunotherapy.

Work is in progress in at least three centres on the estimation of oestrogen and progesterone receptors on mammary tumours in the bitch. In a study of 100 mammary canine tumours it has been found that 37% were positive for oestrogen receptors and 63% were negative (Hamilton et al., 1977). There was no association with the histologic type of tumour and positive or negative results. It is not yet known whether there is any relationship between oestrogen receptor results and therapy in this species. Testosterone implants and drostanalone propionate have been used but no controlled trials are available. It is, however, known in a few cases that there has been no objective regression of metastatic mammary tumours in the lung following androgen therapy.

B. *Prostate*

Carcinoma of the prostate in the dog is a rare condition with a very poor prognosis and there are no records of therapy being tried. Hyperplasia is a very common condition and a reduction in size of the prostate can be obtained by castration or administration of oestrogens—usually by a subcutaneous implant of stilboestrol or hexoestrol. Following overdosage or prolonged dosage of stilboestrol metaplastic changes occur in the prostate and there is again an increase in size.

Hepatoid tumours of the circumanal glands also respond to

oestrogens, but as his is of a temporary nature surgery plus radiotherapy is preferable therapy.

VI. Immunotherapy

Articles on naturally-occurring tumours in domestic animals as models for research in immunology have appeared in *Bull. Wld Hlth Org.* 49, 81–91 and 205–213.

A. *Immunological Status*

Studies made on the immune reactivity in dogs with lymphosarcoma have shown that IgG levels were significantly low and that haemagglutination titres after sheep erythrocyte immunization were suppressed. Response to tuberculin challenge after sensitization with BCG and *in vitro* lymphocyte blastogenesis after stimulation by PHA or allogeneic lymphocytes were deficient. The reticulo-endothelial system function assessed by clearance of bacteriophage from the circulation was impaired. Cellular immunity assessed by skin graft survival was found to be impaired, but 7 of the 15 dogs tested with viable grafts in place for more than 10 days died suddenly (Weiden *et al.*, 1974). In another study survival of whole skin thickness grafts was the same as in control dogs, whereas using the same technique of skin grafting, prolonged survival of grafts occurred in animals made tolerant by injection of donor spleen cells injected when foetuses *in utero* (Owen *et al.*, 1975). The results on skin grafting in these dogs resemble those made in lymphosarcoma in man, whereas in Hodgkins' disease in man skin grafts are frequently prolonged. However, there seems little doubt that dogs with lymphosarcoma can show many deficiencies in immune reactivity as is well recognized in lymphoreticular neoplasia in man.

Using similar tests in dogs with solid tumours these animals were found to be intact with regard to humoral immunity and reticulo-endothelial system function, but had a partial deficit in cellular immune reactivity (Weiden *et al.*, 1974).

In the rather special case of the transmissible venereal tumour (TVT), humoral antibody against membrane-associated antigens has been demonstrated using the indirect membrane immunofluorescence test (Cohen, 1972). Circulating antibody to the tumour, as well as *in vivo* coating of the tumour cells with antibody, could be detected at 40 days or more after transplantation. Anti-TVT activity was centred in the 19S, intermediate S and 7S fractions of the anti-TVT serum and a cross reaction demonstrated between anti-TVT sera of clinical cases occurring in Ireland and Malaya.

In vitro tumour cell cytotoxicity using high numbers of lymphocytes from dogs bearing tumours and the blocking of such reactivity by autologous serum, have been demonstrated by Fidler (1974). Serum from dogs with the same histological type of neoplasm inhibited allogeneic lymphocytotoxicity, while serum from dogs with other tumours or normal dogs did not. Stimulation of tumour growth *in vitro* by low ratios of autochthonous lymphocytes was demonstrated. Furthermore, autologous serum appeared to potentiate the stimulation of tumour growth above a simple blocking effect of lymphocyte-mediated cytotoxicity. The author states that these results confirmed earlier data and supported the hypothesis that the early immune response to neoplasia might directly stimulate rather than inhibit tumour growth.

B. *Spontaneous Regression of Tumours*

As well as regression of known virus-induced papillomas in dogs and cattle and the regressions of fibropapillomas in horses where the aetiology is less certain, regression is well recognized in cutaneous histiocytomas in dogs and in the transmissible venereal tumour of dogs. The canine histiocytoma looks very malignant when examined histologically, but in a detailed study of over 200 cases neither widespread metastases nor death as a result of the tumour were observed (Taylor *et al.*, 1969). The tumours rarely recurred at the site of excision, at a new site or at two sites simultaneously. The malignancy of the transmissible venereal tumour can be very variable, ranging from spontaneous regression to metastasis and death of the host. Complete regression is followed by transplantation immunity (Cohen, 1972).

Unlike the position in man, there appear to be no records of spontaneous regression of renal carcinoma or malignant melanoma in the dog. Neuroblastoma and chorion carcinoma have not been reported in dogs.

C. *Vaccination*

Preventive vaccination is successfully practised against two neoplastic diseases of domestic animals—fibropapillomatosis in cattle and Marek's disease of chickens. In the case of Marek's disease of

chickens which is due to a Herpes virus, a live attenuated virus is used
which does not prevent infection with virulent virus but prevents the
development of neoplasia. The exact mechanism is as yet unknown.
Vaccines free of viral nucleic acids have been prepared and shown to
be effective in prophylaxis (Epstein, 1975). This is an important step
forward in the eventual vaccination against Burkitt's lymphoma
where an attenuated virus cannot be used because of the problem of
excluding residual traces of viral DNA which could induce malignant
transformation.

Research on feline lymphosarcoma virus is particularly relevant to
the human leukaemia problem in view of the recent report on the
infective transmission and characterization of a C-type virus released
by cultured human myeloid leukaemia cells (Teich et al., 1975) and
the isolation of an infectious C-type oncornavirus from human
leukemic bone marrow cells (Nooter et al., 1975).

The ultimate control of feline leukemia and related diseases
would be the development of an FeLV vaccine. Jarrett and his co-
workers (1975) have conducted studies in which cats inoculated with
live feline lymphoblastoid cells of the FL74 line were shown to
develop high titres of antibody to feline oncornavirus-associated cell
membrane antigen (FOCMA). Eight cats were subsequently challenged with a large dose of feline leukemia virus (FeLV) of a highly
pathogenic strain. All resisted infection, while ten cats given only the
challenge virus became infected. The FeLV pro 'uced by FL74 cells
was shown to be of extremely low infectivity in cats and in cultured
feline cells. Cats inoculated with either FL74 cells or virus purified
from them did not become infected. The purified virus did not
induce FOCMA antibody in cats not previously exposed to FeLV.
The fact that FL74 cells are highly immunogenic, but produce virus
of low infectivity, is of value in devising vaccines against FeLV. Cats
were also inoculated with FL74 cells which had been inactivated with
paraformaldehyde. They developed FOMA antibody, reaching a
peak titre of 256, and no virus could be cultured either from the
vaccine preparations or from the tissues of the cats.

D. *Clinical Immunotherapy*

Very few trials of immunotherapy to treat malignant tumours in the
dog and cat have been conducted. Some information on active non-
specific immunotherapy has been obtained in the dog using BCG
intravenously. Following injection of 50,000–250,000 organisms of
dried percutaneous BCG intravenously in dogs, there is usually little

clinical effect, except that in some dogs pyrexia occurs at some period during the following 24 hours and there may be dullness and temporary anorexia. Following more than one injection there may be an anaphylactic-like response and it has been found advisable to inject antihistamine drugs intramuscularly 20–30 minutes before administration of BCG by the intravenous route.

Histopathological changes following injections of BCG are essentially similar in normal dogs and in dogs with spontaneous osteosarcoma (Owen and Bostock, 1974). The most obvious feature in the lungs is a marked perivascular mononuclear reaction, the predominant cell types being macrophages and lymphocytes. Additionally in the lung parenchyma there are small granulomas with a central zone of macrophages surrounded by a thin rim of lymphocytes. In the liver there is an infiltration of the portal connective tissue with mononuclear cells, again with macrophages predominating. The bronchial lymph nodes and tonsils show a marked follicular lymphoid hyperplasia.

In dogs injected intrathoracically with BCG there is a marked response to PPD injected intradermally 4 weeks later, in contrast to the dogs injected intravenously where the response is usually negative. In intrathoracically injected dogs, numerous white granulomata 2–3 mm in diameter occur on the pleura a few weeks after injection.

In 12 dogs with spontaneous osteosarcoma which had no radiographic evidence of lung metastases at the time of clinical examination, the affected limb was amputated and percutaneous BCG injected intravenously at the following time intervals in weeks: 1, 2, 4, 8 followed by injections every 8 weeks to one year. Two dogs are still alive at 35 and 24 weeks. Of the 10 dogs now dead the median survival was 40 weeks. No exact matched controls were available, but 11 dogs in the same Veterinary School also radiographically free of metastases in which the affected limb was amputated and the dogs not given BCG, had a median survival of 14 weeks. The difference between medians is significant at $P < 0.01$. In two long-term survivors (65 weeks) which had not received BCG for 2 or more months before death, granulomas were not present on post-mortem examination. More observations are in progress to determine if granulomas in liver and lung heal in time in all dogs which have been injected with BCG (Owen and Bostock, 1975).

In contrast to the promising results with osteosarcoma in which there was no evidence of enhancement and a probable delay in the appearance of metastases, the results of chemotherapy followed by intravenous BCG injection in dogs with spontaneous lymphosarcoma have been poor. Following quadruple therapy of vincristine, cytosine arabinoside, cyclophosphamide and prednisone, dogs have been given BCG intravenously alone or mixed with living allogenic lymphosarcoma cells. In all 16 dogs so far given this therapy, rapid relapse (1-2 weeks) has occurred, whereas dogs maintained on chemotherapy have had a mean survival time of 6 months. Lymph nodes in most of these dogs given BCG have again regressed following a second course of chemotherapy. Because of the impaired immunity of these dogs and the immunosuppressive effect of the drugs, especially cyclophosphamide and prednisone, it seems unlikely that modifications of this approach would be any more successful. Dogs with lymphosarcoma given chemotherapy and then injected with BCG appear to react with considerably less granulomata than do normal dogs and this observation is also undergoing further study. Trials with BCG in other malignant tumours, particularly following excision of malignant mammary tumours in the bitch, are in progress and are showing similar results to those obtained with orteosarcoma.

References

Betton, G. R. (1975). "The Biology and Immunology of Canine Melanoma". Ph.D. Thesis, University of Cambridge.

Bostock, D. E. (1973). *J. Small Anim. Pract.* **14**, 27–41.

Bostock, D. E. (1975). *Europ. J. Cancer*, **11**, 389–396.

Bostock, D. E., Owen, L. N., Onions, D. E. and Theilin, G. H. (1975). Personal observation.

Cohen, Dan (1972). *Int. J. Cancer*, **10**, 207–212.

Cohen, Dan (1973). *Europ. J. Cancer*, **9**, 253–258.

Cohen, D. and Steel, G. G. (1972). *Br. J. Cancer*, **26**, 413–419.

Dorn, C. R., Taylor, D. O. N., Frye, F. L. and Hibbard, H. H. (1968a). *J. Natl. Cancer Inst.* **40**, 295–305.

Dorn, C. R., Taylor, D. O. N., Schneider, R., Hibbard, H. H. and Klauber, M. R. (1968b). *J. Natl. Cancer Inst.* **40**, 307–318.

Epstein, M. A. (1975). *Nature*, **253**, 6–7.

Fidler, I. J. (1974). *Fed. Proc.* **33**/3, 615.

Freireich, E. J., Gehan, E. A., Rall, D. P., Schmidt, L. H. and Skipper, H. E. (1966). *Cancer Chemother. Rept.* **50**, 219–244.

Fraumeni, J. F. (1967). *Cancer N. Y.* **20**, 967–973.

Hamilton, J. M., Else, R. W. and Forshaw, P. (1977). *Vet. Rec.* **101**, 258–260.

Hampe, J. F. and Misdorp, W. (1974). *Bull. Wld Hlth Org.* **50**, 111–133.

Hayden, D. W. and Nielsen, S. W. (1971). *J. Small Anim. Pract.* **12**, 687–698.

Hill, R. and Dumas, K. (1973). *In* "Pharmacological Models in Contraceptive Development." WHO, Karolinska Institut Stockholm, p. 74–83.

Jarrett, W., Jarrett, O., Mackey, L., Laird, N., Hood, C. and Hay, D. (1975). *Int. J. Cancer*, **16**, 135–141.

Lombard, L. S., Moloney, J. B. and Rickard, G. C. (1963). *Ann. N. Y. Acad. Sci.* **108**, 1086–1105.

Mackey, L. J., Jarrett, W. F. H., Jarrett, O. and Laird, Helen M. (1972). *J. Natl. Cancer Inst.* **48**, 1663–1670.

Newton, K. A. (1974). Personal communication.

Nooter, K., Aarssen, A. M., Bentvelzen, P., De Groot, F. G. and Van Pelt, F. G. (1975). *Nature, Lond.* **256**, 595–597.

Owen, L. N. (1962). *Brit. J. Cancer*, **16**, 441–452.

Owen, L. N. (1964). *Brit. J. Cancer*, **18**, 407–418.

Owen, L. N. and Nielsen, S. W. (1968). *Europ. J. Cancer*, **4**, 391–393.

Owen, L. N. (1969a). *Europ. J. Cancer*, **5**, 615–618.

Owen, L. N. (1969b). *In* "Bone Tumours in Man and Animals", pp. 29–52. Butterworths, London.

Owen, L. N. and Steel, G. G. (1969). *Brit. J. Cancer*, **23**, 493–509.

Owen, L. N. (1971). *Europ. J. Cancer*, **7**, 525–528.

Owen, L. N. (1972). Unpublished observations.

Owen, L. N. (1973). *In* "Bone: Certain Aspects of Neoplasia" (C. H. G. Price and F. G. M. Ross, eds), pp. 327–334. Butterworths, London.

Owen, L. N. and Bostock, D. E. (1973). *Europ. J. Cancer*, **9**, 747–752.

Owen, L. N. and Bostock, D. E. (1974). *Europ. J. Cancer*, **10**, 775–780.

Owen, L. N. and Bostock, D. E. (1975). Unpublished observations.

Owen, L. N., Bostock, D. E. and Halliwell, R. E. W. (1975). *Europ J. Cancer*, **11**, 187–191.

Owen, L. N. and Morgan, D. R. (1975). *J. Europ. Cancer*. In press.

Peperzeel, van H. A. (1972). *In* "Patterns of Tumour Growth after Irradiation" (1970), pp. 34–40. Drukkerij van Denderen, Groningen.

Post, J. E., Noronha, F. and Rickard, C. G. (1969). *Comp. Leuk. Res. Bibl. Haemat.* **36**. (R. M. Dutcher, ed.). Karger, Basel 1970.

Priester, W. A., and Mantel, N. (1971). *J. Natl. Cancer Inst.* **47**, 1333–1344.

Ravdin, R. E., Lewison, E. F. and Slack, N. H. (1970). *Surg. Gynaecol. Obstet.* **131**, 1055–1064.

Roga, V., Hedeman, I. P. and Olson, B. H. (1971). *Cancer Chemother. Rpt.* **55**, 101–113.

Schneider, R., Dorn, C. R. and Taylor, D. O. N. (1969). *J. Natl. Cancer Inst.*, **43**, 1249–1261.

Silver, I. A. (1972). *J. Small Anim. Pract* **13**, 351–358.

Snyder, S. R. and Theilen, G. H. (1969). *Nature, Lond.* **221**, 1074–1075.

Squire, R. A. and Bush, M. (1973). *In* "Unifying Concepts of Leukemia". *Bibl. Haemat.* **39**. (R. M. Dutcher and L. Chieco-Bianchi, eds), p. 189. Basel.

Stjernswärd, J. (1974). *Lancet*, **2**, 1285–1286.

Taylor, D. O. N., Dorn, C. R. and Luis, O. H. (1969). *Cancer Res.* **29**, 83–89.

Teich, N. M., Weiss, R. A., Salahuddin, S. Z., Gallagher, R. E., Gillespie, D. H. and Gallo, R. C. (1975). *Nature, Lond.* **256**, 551–555.

Weiden, P. L., Storb, R., Kolb, H.-J., Ocho, H. D., Graham, T. C., Tsoi, M.-S., Schroeder, M.-L. and Thomas, E. D. (1974). *J. Natl. Cancer Inst.* **53**, 1049–1056.

Weijer, K., Head, K. W., Misdorp, W. and Hampe, J. F. (1972). *J. Natl. Cancer Inst.* **49**, 1697–1704.

Chapter VI

Immunology and Immunotherapy of Experimental and Clinical Metastases

M. · V. PIMM AND R. W. BALDWIN

Cancer Research Campaign Laboratories, The University, University Park, Nottingham, England

I. Introduction

Immunological factors are now thought to play a role in modifying or even controlling malignant disease. This concept has developed firstly from well-substantiated investigations showing that many experimentally-induced animal tumours exhibit neoantigens which are recognized by the host and this leads to the induction of immune rejection responses against the tumour (Baldwin, 1973; Herberman, 1976). Secondly, human studies have reached the stage where *in vitro* tests for tumour immune reactions, initially developed with well-defined animal systems, have been shown to be positive with a wide range of human tumour types (Hellström and Hellström, 1974; Baldwin and Embleton, 1977). This indicates that many human tumours express neoantigens which elicit an immune response in the patient, although there is considerable controversy as to whether these function to produce potential tumour rejection (Baldwin, 1975; Herberman and Oldham, 1975; Baldwin and Embleton, 1977). Nevertheless, the evidence from experimental studies is now overwhelmingly in support of the view that immunological factors are important in the tumour-host relationship and it is pertinent to consider their role in controlling metastatic spread of tumours. Before considering the special case of the immunology of metastatic tumours, it is necessary to broadly outline the concepts of tumour immunology.

The currently accepted concept that many tumours express immunologically recognizable determinants, defined as tumour-associated antigens, is derived basically from transplantation studies in which tumours induced which chemical carcinogens or oncogenic viruses in animals of highly inbred (syngeneic) strains can be transplanted into other members of the same strain so as to exclude the development of immune responses against normal tissue transplantation antigens. Employing these model systems it has been established that hosts *pre-immunized* in a variety of ways against tumour cells are protected against a subsequent challenge with cells of the immunizing tumour (Baldwin, 1973; Herberman, 1976). For example, surgical resection of a developing subcutaneous tumour graft often provides complete protection against a subsequent contralateral challenge with cells of the resected tumour. Tumour immunity can also be induced by immunization with tumour cells attenuated so as to prevent their continuous growth, e.g. by X-irradiation, and this form of immunization can be enhanced by including so-called "immunological adjuvants" such as bacillus Calmette Guérin (BCG) in the treatment protocol (McKhann and Gunnarsson, 1974). This immunity can generally be transferred from immune donors with lymphoid cells, e.g. lymph node lymphocytes, and it is generally accepted that cell mediated immunity is primarily important in immunological rejection of tumours. The role of tumour specific antibody is more problematical, since contradictory effects have been obtained when attempting to transfer immunity against transplanted tumour cells with serum from tumour immune donors. Weak suppression of tumour growth or, quite frequently, no significant effect was observed. In some cases, passively transferred serum even produced enhancement of tumour growth suggesting that tumour specific antibody plays no significant role in tumour rejection. This view is now thought to be too extreme, however, since antibody may produce a cytotoxic effect either through fixation of complement or probably more effectively through cooperation with normal lymphoid cells, i.e. cell-dependent antibody killing (Forman and Möller, 1973).

Experimental animal studies have also established that hosts with a tumour developing at one site which is beyond immunological control can, nevertheless, reject a concomitant challenge with cells of the same tumour implanted at a contralateral site, providing that the challenge inoculum is not too large (Gershon et al., 1967; Howell et al., 1975). For example, mice bearing subcutaneous grafts of transplanted sarcomas were found to reject a contralateral challenge with cells of the same tumour (Chandradasa, 1973; Vaage, 1973). This tumour specific immune response was directed specifically against the tumour associated antigens of the primary tumour graft, since growths of contralateral challenges with different tumours were not inhibited. It should also be noted that the capacity of the tumour-bearing host to reject the second tumour challenge waned as the primary tumour increased in size (eclipse phenomenon) but resistance was restored following resection of the primary tumour (Le François et al., 1971; Vaage, 1973; Howell et al., 1975). These studies on concomitant immunity indicate that the tumour bearing host does, in many instances, develop a systemic immune response which is capable of rejecting tumour cells implanted at a distant site and this is highly relevant in considering the role of immunological factors in controlling metastatic tumour deposits.

The studies briefly reviewed above indicate that experimental animal tumours may be subject to host immunological control, but this depends upon the tumour in question expressing tumour associated rejection antigens. In this context, it should be recognized that not all tumours have this type of neoantigen, e.g. carcinogen-induced mammary carcinomas in the rat (Baldwin and Embleton, 1974). Furthermore, it should be appreciated that the frequency of expression of tumour rejection antigens on naturally occurring (spontaneous) animal tumours is much lower than that observed with tumours deliberately induced with extrinsic agents, such as chemical carcinogens or oncogenic viruses (Baldwin, 1973). This point has not received sufficient emphasis but it is clearly important in equating concepts developed with experimental animal tumours to human malignant disease. Here the evidence for tumour associated antigens is still largely circumstantial or has been derived from *in vitro* studies of tumour immune reactions, and so cannot firmly be correlated with tumour rejection (Baldwin and Embleton, 1977; Herberman, 1976).

II. Role of Immunity in Control of Metastases

Immunological factors clearly play a role in the growth of localized deposits of experimental tumours. In addition, there is considerable evidence to support the view that similar mechanisms may operate in the tumour-bearing host to control metastatic spread of experimental tumours. This evidence has been derived from observations on tumour specific transplantation resistance to metastasis both in tumour bearer and tumour immune animals. Conversely a positive increase in the degree or extent of metastatic spread is often observed in animals receiving immunosuppressive therapy. For a review on the role of immunodepression in malignancy (*see* Stutman, 1975).

A. *Facilitation of Metastases by Immunosuppression*

Much of the evidence for immunological control of metastases comes from experimental studies on the influence of immunosuppressive treatments on the propensity of tumours to metastasise. Immunosuppression by procedures such as whole body X-irradiation, thymectomy or treatment with anti-lymphocyte or anti-thymocyte globulin has been reported by many workers to encourage tumour dissemination (Table 1). For example, in studies with the syngeneically transplanted Lewis lung carcinoma in C57B1 mice, James and Salsbury (1974) found that treatment of mice bearing subcutaneous grafts with heterologous rabbit anti-mouse thymocyte globulin significantly increased the numbers of pulmonary metastases, compared to animals treated with normal rabbit globulin. There was, however, no influence on the rate of growth of the initial subcutaneous tumour. This facilitation of metastasis was associated with an early release of tumour cells into the blood, this being attributed to the failure of draining lymph nodes to respond to the tumour. This lack of lymph node responsiveness was seen as a failure to release large pyroninophilic immunoblasts into the efferent lymph. These immunoblasts are normally released in large numbers into the lymph draining tumour sites (Alexander *et al.*, 1969) reaching a peak four days after tumour implantation in the case of the Lewis lung tumour. In anti-thymocyte globulin treated mice, the

TABLE 1

Facilitation of metastasis of transplanted animal tumours by immunosuppression

Species	Primary Tumour Type	Site	Immunosuppressive treatment	Increased metastases to:	Author
Rat	MCA-induced sarcoma	Subcutaneous	Anti-lymphocyte serum	Omentum and mesentery	Fisher et al. (1969b)
Rat	BP-induced sarcoma	Intramuscular	Whole body irradiation or prolonged thoracic duct drainage	Lung and lymph nodes	Eccles and Alexander (1975)
Rat	Yoshida ascites sarcoma	Intramuscular	Whole body irradiation	Lung	Van den Brenk et al. (1971)
Hamster	Lymphoma	Subcutaneous	Anti-lymphocyte serum	Axillary, mediastinal and perirenal lymph nodes	Gershon and Carter (1970)
Mouse	Lewis lung carcinoma	Subcutaneous	Anti-thymocyte serum	Lungs	James and Salsbury (1974)
Mouse	Lewis lung carcinoma	Subcutaneous	Irradiation, or neonatal thymectomy, or thymectomy and irradiation	Lungs	Carnaud et al. (1974)
Mouse	Alveolar cell carcinoma	Subcutaneous	Whole body irradiation or hydrocortisone treatment	Lungs	Yuhas and Pazmiño (1974)
Mouse	Mammary carcinoma	Subcutaneous	Anti-lymphocyte serum	Lungs and liver	Fisher et al. (1969a)
Mouse	Lymphoma	Intradermal	Thymectomy	Liver, kidney	Weston et al. (1974)
Mouse	Sarcoma 180	Dorsum of foot	Thymectomy and/or anti-lymphocyte serum	Draining and distant lymph nodes	Isbister et al. (1971) Deodhar and Crile (1969)

failure of immunoblast release was paralleled precisely by the appearance of circulating tumour cells, which normally did not become apparent until the tumour had been *in situ* for ten days. The earlier release of potentially metastatic tumour cells from sub-cutaneous growths under anti-thymocyte globulin treatment was also indicated by the ultimate appearance of pulmonary metastases in treated mice from which small, i.e. less than eight-day-old, sub-cutaneous tumours had been surgically excised. Normally, no pulmonary metastases would be produced in animals from which such small tumours had been removed.

Increased incidence of pulmonary metastases from the Lewis lung carcinoma by immunosuppression was also reported by Carnaud *et al.* (1974). Here immunosuppression by whole body γ-irradiation, adult thymectomy and irradiation, or neonatal thymectomy, significantly increased the numbers of lung metastases from subcutaneous growths as compared with intact controls. Immunological restoration of mice by injection of lymphoid cells, or thymus reimplantation, reduced significantly the numbers of metastases when compared with unrestored animals. In keeping with the observations of James and Salsbury (1974), immunological impairment had a more pronounced effect on metastases than upon the initial tumour implant, suggesting that host immune responses might even be more efficient with disseminated tumour foci than with a single localized tumour mass.

Confirmation of the increased incidence of metastases in immunosuppressed animals has been reported with a number of other experimental tumour systems (Table 1), including those with propensities to metastasise to other anatomical sites besides the lungs. For example, Gershon and Carter (1970) found that anti-lymphocyte serum treatment encouraged metastases to axillary, mediastinal and perirenal lymph nodes in hamsters bearing a subcutaneously transplanted lymphoma, while thymectomy encouraged hepatic and renal metastases from a transplanted mouse lymphoma (Weston *et al.*, 1974).

In many of the above instances, the facilitation of metastases was not accompanied by an increased rate of growth of the primary tumour, suggesting that immunological factors may play a more decisive role in the control of disseminated rather than localized tumours. Indeed, Yuhas and Pazmiño (1974) reported that, while metastases of a transplanted alveolar cell carcinoma were encouraged by immunosuppression, this treatment significantly retarded growth of the initial subcutaneous tumour graft. This retardation of localized tumours by immunosuppression has been described with several tumour types (Prehn, 1969; Spärck, 1969; Yuhas *et al.*, 1974), and has led Prehn and Lappé (1971) to argue that weak immunological responses can, under certain circumstances, positively encourage local tumour development (*see* also Prehn, 1976).

There is some evidence that immunosuppression in man, too, may encourage metastases from primary tumours (Stutman, 1975). It has been well documented that long term immunosuppression in, for example, patients receiving renal allografts, is accompanied by an increase in malignant disease, particularly lymphoma (Penn, 1974). If these lesions show any unusual propensity to metastasize, a relationship in man between prolonged immunosuppression and enhanced metastases may well emerge and Penn (1974) has described a group of patients with pre-existing malignancies receiving organ transplants and maintained on immunosuppression in whom residual tumour grew at "spectacular rates" with metastatic deposits even in the homografts themselves.

B. *Induction of Transplantation Resistance to "Metastatic" Challenge*

Many of the initial experimental observations on the induction of tumour transplantation resistance were made with localized subcutaneous or intramuscular tumour cell challenges into animals immunized by surgical removal of localized tumours, or receiving local injections of irradiated malignant tissue. There are, however, many more recent reports indicating that this type of tumour immunity may operate systemically, and may even be stronger than at the subcutaneous or intramuscular sites. In some instances, also, a positive facilitation of growth of disseminated tumour challenge inocula is observed in conventionally immune animals, although this enhancement too, probably has an immunological basis. Vaage *et al.* (1971) working with 3-methylcholanthrene-induced mouse sarcomas, demonstrated transplantation resistance to intravenous and intraportal challenges, tumours developing mainly in the lungs and liver respectively in untreated control animals. Resistance, as measured by the maximum tumour inoculum rejected, was greater to an intravenous or intraportal challenge than to challenges subcutaneously or intraperitoneally, and it was concluded that tumour rejection responses in some organs, particularly in the liver, could be more effective than in others, probably explaining the predilection of some organs to develop metastases. Intra-arterial challenges of tumour immune mice demonstrated resistance at several other anatomical sites, including kidneys, ovaries and adrenal glands. The immunological nature of the suppression of tumours throughout the body was indicated by the passive transfer of immunity to disseminated challenges with lymph node cells from tumour immune donors. These findings have been confirmed by Milas *et al.* (1974a) who similarly found immunological resistence to artificial pulmonary metastases, produced by the intravenous injection of cells, in C3Hf/BV mice. This immunity to disseminated challenge was directed specifically against cells of the tumour used to immunize the challenged animals, and could be passively transferred by spleen or lymph node cells from immune donors.

In contrast to these reports, Wexler *et al.* (1972, 1975) demonstrated that prior immunization against carcinogen-induced sarcomas in C57B1 mice significantly enhanced the growth of pulmonary metastases. This effect was most pronounced with tumours which were highly immunogenic, as defined by the maximum cell numbers rejected subcutaneously in immunized animals, and these authors suggested that cells from highly immunogenic tumours entering the circulation are less likely to be destroyed than if they remained at extra-vascular sites. It was also suggested that this facilitation of metastatic growth might be attributable to the effect of circulating blocking factors (*see* page 178). In contrast to the encouragement of metastases from the highly immunogenic sarcomas, tumours with lower immunogenic potential were controlled when injected intravenously into pre-immunized animals, and a non-immunogenic sarcoma grew in the lungs in the same manner in normal and pre-treated hosts (Wexler *et al.*, 1975). In support of the concept that humoral blocking factors might facilitate protection of circulating malignant cells against immunological rejection, Milas and Mujagic (1973) reported that splenectomy greatly reduced the number of pulmonary metastases in mice receiving intravenous tumour cell inocula of a 3-methylcholanthrene-induced sarcoma. The spleen is known to be the major antibody-producing organ (Rowley, 1950), and its removal has been shown to decrease levels of circulating anti-tumour antibody (Möller, 1965), and the level of serum blocking factor capable of protecting tumour cells from *in vitro* lymphocyte mediated cytotoxicity (Hellström *et al.*, 1970).

C. *Concomitant Immunity to Metastases in Tumour Bearing Hosts*

In addition to the demonstration of transplantation resistance to localized and, more particularly, disseminated tumour cell challenges in pre-immunized animals, the most direct experimental evidence for immunological control of metastases comes from observations on concomitant immunity. This, as already indicated, is the ability of an animal bearing an established and progressively growing tumour to resist a further challenge with the same tumour at another site. This form of immunity has been described with mouse mammary carcinomas (Fisher *et al.*, 1970) and rat and mouse sarcomas (Fisher *et al.*, 1970; Deckers *et al.*, 1973), SV40 virus-induced tumours in mice (Zarling and Tevethia, 1973), and lymphoma in hamsters (Gershon *et al.*, 1967) (Table 2). In these tests artificial metastases of subcutaneous tumour cell inocula, capable of initiating progressive growth in untreated control animals were rejected in animals with already established tumour deposits. In some cases only limited cell numbers were controlled in tumour bearing animals, but this concomitant immunity could, nevertheless, play a potential role in protecting against disseminating metastases. Thus in comparable studies with 3-methylcholanthrene-induced sarcomas in mice, Milas *et al.* (1974a) demonstrated specific concomitant immunity to artificial pulmonary metastases, produced by intravenously injected

TABLE 2

Concomitant immunity against secondary tumour deposits in animals with established tumour growths

Species	Tumour type	Primary site	Secondary deposit		Author
			Site	No. cells rejected	
Hamster	Lymphoblastic lymphoma	Subcutaneous	Subcutaneous	1×10^8	Gershon *et al.* (1967)
Mouse	Mammary carcinoma	Subcutaneous	Subcutaneous	1×10^4	Fisher *et al.* (1970)
Mouse	SV40-transformed kidney cells	Subcutaneous	Subcutaneous	5×10^6	Zarling and Tevethia (1973)
Mouse	MCA-induced sarcoma	Subcutaneous	Subcutaneous	1×10^3	Deckers *et al.* (1973)
Mouse	MCA-induced sarcoma	Subcutaneous	Lungs[a]	1×10^5	Milas *et al.* (1974a)
Rat	MCA-induced sarcoma	Subcutaneous	Lungs[a]	2×10^5	Fisher *et al.* (1970)
Rat	MCA-induced sarcoma	Subcutaneous	Subcutaneous	1×10^6	Pimm and Baldwin (1976d)

[a] Pulmonary deposit produced by intravenous injection of cells.

cells, in mice bearing subcutaneously established tumour grafts of the same sarcoma. This protection against disseminating tumour was most marked when the initial tumour had grown for 14 days, suggesting that maximum host sensitization was necessary before concomitant control of metastases could be fully effective. In keeping with this suggestion that full host sensitization is necessary to generate concomitant immunity, Gershon et al. (1968), studying hamster lymphomas, found that removal of the initial tumour graft only 7 days after implantation led to a decrease in immunity, whereas animals with more established initial tumours showed marked concomitant immunity to subcutaneous challenge. Furthermore, surgical removal of 7-day-old tumours was followed by overt appearance of metastases, although such metastases were never found in animals killed with larger tumour growths, although viable tumour cells are demonstrable in blood and lymph nodes of such animals.

In addition to the observation that concomitant immunity generated by initial localized tumour deposits may protect against distant localized or disseminated metastases, there is also evidence to suggest that metastatic deposits themselves may influence the growth of the initial tumour mass. Thus with the transplantable alveolar cell carcinoma in the mouse, Yuhas et al. (1974) demonstrated that subsequent growth of subcutaneous tumours was retarded if the animal also received a simultaneous intravenous injection of live, but not dead, tumour cells. These intravenously injected cells produced multiple tumour deposits in the lungs, but there was no difference in the growth of these artificial metastases between animals with or without a subcutaneous tumour growth. That is, there was no concomitant immunity generated by the subcutaneous tumour against the pulmonary metastases, but the metastases were capable of influencing the growth of the primary tumour. These experiments differ from those of Milas et al. (1974a), however, in that cells were injected intravenously, to produce artificial metastases in the lungs at the same time as the animal received subcutaneous tumour growths, and it could be argued from the observation of Milas et al. (1974a) that animals had not had sufficient time to generate concomitant immunity stimulated by the subcutaneous growth.

D. *Role of Draining Lymph Nodes in Controlling Early Spread of Tumour*

While systemic immune responses can clearly control the progress of potentially metastatic tumour cells, other studies have shown that the anti-tumour activity of lymph nodes draining the site of a primary tumour might be more important in controlling tumour dissemination early in tumour growth and before systemic tumour immunity has fully developed. Thus in tests with a transplanted mouse sarcoma (S180) Crile (1968) has shown in a series of experiments that in contrast to tumour immunity induced by surgical removal of tumour alone, removal of regional (popliteal) lymph nodes together with the tumour, after the latter had been *in situ* for only 4 to 10 days, did not leave the animal immune to further tumour challenge. In contrast removal of draining nodes after 10 days, by which time systemic immunity had developed, did not influence the expression of subsequent host immunity. Most importantly, removal of draining nodes early in tumour growth, before or at the same time as tumour removal led to an increased incidence and severity of metastases and it was concluded that such draining nodes were important in the host's early control of tumour dissemination. Lymphoreticular reactions and immune responses in lymph nodes draining the site of tumour growth are discussed in detail in *Chapter II*.

III. Failure of Immunological Control of Metastases

Immunological defences can inhibit growth of both localized and metastatic tumour deposits, but this control in many cases breaks down or at best is ineffective in the tumour-bearing host. Several explanations have been proposed to account for this failure of immunological control including:

    A. "Sneaking through"
    B. Alterations in neoantigen expression and/or function
    C. Malfunction of the immune system.

The last interpretation is currently viewed as being especially important, but it is likely that all these processes take place in the tumour-bearing host and these may influence the metastatic capacity of tumours.

A. *"Sneaking Through"*

The "sneaking through" hypothesis implies that a nascent tumour may not initially provide a sufficient stimulus to induce an effective immune response so that when host defences are eventually mobilized, the tumour is already at a size which is beyond immunological control

(Old and Boyse, 1964). This explanation may seem trivial and has been referred to by Klein (1975) as a "numbers game" rather than a specific mechanism. Nevertheless, it may be important especially with tumours where there is an early metastatic spread. For example, cells are rapidly released from subcutaneous grafts of a transplanted rat epithelioma so that even when the primary implant was surgically resected within ten days of transplantation, a high proportion of the animals developed pulmonary metastases (Baldwin and Pimm, 1973a). In comparison, cytotoxic lymphoid cells were not detected in regional nodes until two weeks after subcutaneous inoculation of viable tumour cells, and only later was it possible to demonstrate reactivity in lymphocytes taken from para-aortic nodes, spleen or blood (Flannery *et al.*, 1973).

B. *Alterations in Neoantigen Expression and/or Function*

Tumour cells undoubtedly show marked variations in the degree of neoantigen expression, so that whilst a tumour may provoke an effective immunological response, subpopulations of cells may not be susceptible to immune rejection. This deficiency in neoantigen expression may result from *quantitative changes*, the tumour cells lacking effective levels of tumour antigen. Alternatively the defect may be *functional*, so that whilst neoantigens continue to be expressed upon the tumour cell, they become inappropriate targets for rejections mediated either by sensitized lymphoid cells or tumour specific antibody.

Variability in neoantigen expression even amongst tumours induced with a single agent has been well documented (Baldwin, 1973; Baldwin and Price, 1975). For example, transplanted murine sarcomas originally induced with chemical carcinogens such as 3-methylchol-anthrene exhibited a wide range of immunogenicities, some readily inducing specific rejection responses when transplanted into synge-netic hosts, whilst others were practically non-immunogenic (Bartlett, 1972). Accordingly it is to be expected that primary tumours may be composed of cell populations expressing widely different amounts of neoantigen. This has been demonstrated in at least one study with 3-methylcholanthrene-induced murine sarcomas where sub-lines were established by transplanting into syngeneic mice tissue taken from two opposite poles of the primary tumour (Prehn, 1970). These were then examined for their capacity to elicit tumour immunity following surgical resection of developing tumour grafts. At least one pair of tumour sub-lines were shown to express different tumour rejection antigens implying the presence of mixed tumour cell populations in the primary tumour. Other pairs of tumour sub-lines, while not showing complete antigenic differences, often exhibited variations in immunogenic potential.

Neoantigen expression has also been shown, in some cases, to be cell cycle dependent, with maximal and minimal expression in the G_1 and S period respectively (Nicolson, 1976). For example Cikes and Klein (1972) showed that the expression of cell surface antigens on Moloney virus-induced lymphoma cells in the S phase was approximately a third to a half of that on G_1 phase cells. These studies also indicated that tumour antigen expression on lymphoma cells was inversely related to their growth rate and this may be relevant to escape of dormant metastatic tumour deposits from immunological control.

Because of the present limited knowledge on the immunobiology of tumour associated antigens, it is generally assumed that changes in immunogenic potential can be ascribed to quantitative variations in neoantigen expression. It is possible, however, that this variability may reflect *functional* modifications of neoantigens so that they are either unable to provoke tumour rejection responses or, alternatively, the cell surface antigens may not be appropriate receptors for either sensitized lymphoid cells or cytotoxic antibody. One factor important in this context may be the degree of integration of tumour antigens in the cell surface membrane, since this will affect their capacity to function as targets in immune cytolytic reactions. In addition, released tumour antigens may provoke immune responses which are ineffective in causing tumour rejection and these products are also likely to interfere with the functioning of any existing cell mediated immunity towards the tumour (*see* page 178). This is illustrated by studies on the capacity of neoantigens on carcinogen-induced and spontaneous rat tumours, e.g. sarcomas and mammary carcinomas, to elicit immunity against transplanted tumour cells. The tumour rejection antigens associated with these tumours are well integrated components of the cell surface membrane, only being released following degradation extraction procedures such as papain digestion or treatment with 3M KC1 (Baldwin and Price, 1975). Almost all of these tumour types also exhibit other neoantigens, which can be identified as re-expressed embryonic products by their interaction *in vitro* with lymphoid cells or antibody from multiparous pregnant rats (Baldwin et al., 1974a). But the tumour associated embryonic antigens do not necessarily function as rejection antigens. For example, a high proportion of carcinogen-induced and spontaneously arising mammary carcinomas were found to be ineffective in producing transplantation immunity in normal rats against challenge with cells of the immunizing tumour, despite the finding that these tumours had detectable cell surface embryonic antigens capable of producing specific immune responses (Baldwin *et al.*, 1974a). Why these tumour associated embryonic antigens are ineffective in producing tumour rejection has still to be answered, but one relevant factor seems to be that these products are much less well integrated components of the tumour cell surface (Baldwin and Price, 1975). In this context, it should be noted that tumour antigens are released by many tumour cells (Nicolson, 1976) and as discussed later, the capacity to shed or release these products may correlate with metastatic potential (Currie and Alexander, 1974; Kim *et al.*, 1975).

1. *Tumour immunogenicity and metastatic spread*

The proposal that metastasising tumour cells may be deficient in tumour associated rejection antigens and so are not subject to host immunological control is supported by a number of studies showing a correlation between metastasis and tumour immunogenicity. For example, Kim (1970) reported that chemically-induced rat mammary carcinomas which metastasise readily to lymph nodes, lungs and liver following implantation into mammary pads, were not able to evoke tumour immunity when implanted in various ways into normal syngeneic rats. Similarly in other studies with carcinogen-induced rat hepatomas and sarcomas, it was shown that tumours with low immunogenic potential, again defined by transplantation tests, exhibited the greatest tendency for metastatic spread (Proctor *et al.*, 1974). One sarcoma, Mc1 which did not metastasise from intramuscular implants, was highly immunogenic, rats pre-immunized against this tumour rejecting challenges with as many as 2×10^7 tumour cells. In comparison, another sarcoma, Mc3, which readily metastasised to the lungs following intramuscular implantation was not demonstrably immunogenic, producing no resistance to challenge with as few as 10^2 tumour cells.

Relevant to the argument that metastases may be formed in some instances by spread of tumour cells deficient in tumour rejection antigens and therefore not so susceptible to immunological control, there are a number of reports showing differences in immunogenicity between primary animal tumours and metastatic deposits (Deichman and Kluchareva, 1966; Hammond *et al.*, 1968; Goldman *et al.*, 1974; Sugarbaker and Cohen, 1972; Sugarbaker *et al.*, 1971; Faraci, 1974). This is illustrated by the studies of Sugarbaker and Cohen (1972) where tumour lines were established by transplanting into syngeneic mice individual pulmonary tumour nodules from donors bearing grafts of a 3-methylcholanthrene-induced sarcoma. The immunological properties of these established tumour lines was then evaluated by studying their capacity to induce tumour immune rejection responses following surgical resection of developing tumours. Altogether seven tumour lines established from pulmonary tumours were studied and of these, only two were found to express the same tumour rejection antigen as that exhibited by the primary tumour. In these two examples, immunization of mice with tumour derived initially from a pulmonary growth produced protection to challenge with cells of the immunizing pulmonary tumour line as well as the original primary tumour. Two other metastases were also immunogenic in that it was possible to induce immunity against these tumour lines. But in this case, they were found to exhibit tumour antigens different from the primary tumour. Finally, three of the tumour lines derived from metastases did not show any significant immunogenicity when assayed in the tumour transplantation system.

In addition to the transplantation tests, attempts have been made to differentiate between the immunogenicity of primary and metastatic tumour deposits from 3-methylcholanthrene-induced murine sarcomas by the *in vitro* susceptibility to sensitized lymphocytes (Faraci, 1974). In this case, it was found that lymphocytes from mice immunized against the primary tumour recognized the primary tumour as well as cells from two tumour lines (MCA-M1 and MCA-M2) established from pulmonary metastases. Similarly, lymphocytes sensitized against cells from one metastatic line MCA-M1 also reacted with all three target cells. But line MCA-M2 cells did not appear to share antigens with the other two target cells.

The introduction of *in vitro* methods for mapping tumour associated antigens, such as lymphocyte cytotoxicity tests for cell mediated immunity, provide relatively reproducible methods for evaluating tumour antigens on primary tumours and metastatic deposits. Further studies in this area should, therefore, substantiate whether modification of tumour cell surface antigens is an important factor in the metastatic process.

2. Degree of host infiltration of tumour tissue and metastatic spread
The degree of host cell infiltration of tumour varies markedly between tumour types, and clinically tumours with heavy infiltration carry a better prognosis than similar tumours with little infiltration. Experimentally, transplanted animal tumours show a wide range of host cell infiltration (Evans, 1972; Van Loveren and Den Otter, 1974; Szymaniec and James, 1976) and a number of workers have

demonstrated that tumours with poor local host responses show the greater propensity to metastasise. For examples, Eccles and Alexander (1974) with a range of six rat sarcomas found that tumours of low immunogenic potential, capable of eliciting transplantation resistance to only $1 \times 10^3 - 2 \times 10^4$ cells had a low host macrophage infiltration (about 10% of the total cells) and produced metastases in all animals following surgical removal. In contrast, highly immunogenic tumours (eliciting transplantation resistance up to 5×10^7 cells) showed a much greater degree of host infiltration (up to 60% macrophages) and only rarely produced metastases.

C. *Malfunction of the Immune System*

Failure of immune responses in the tumour-bearing host to control tumour growth may result from the intervention of humoral factors which diminish the effectiveness of cell mediated immunity (Hellström and Hellström, 1974; Baldwin and Robins, 1975, 1976, 1977). This concept originally formulated by the Hellströms in terms of circulating "blocking factors" which interact with tumour cells so preventing their recognition by sensitized lymphoid cells, is based upon the demonstration that the *in vitro* cytotoxicity of lymphoid cells from tumour-bearing donors for tumour cells can be specifically abrogated by treatment of target cells with tumour-bearer serum. Since the original description of tumour-bearer serum blocking of lymph node cell cytotoxicity for Moloney virus-induced murine sarcomas (Hellström and Hellström, 1969), this phenomenon has been demonstrated with many experimental animal and human tumours (Hellström and Hellström, 1974; Baldwin and Robins, 1975). Interference with cell mediated immunity in the tumour-bearing host can operate, however, through several pathways. These include *blocking* of tumour antigen at the cell surface following interaction with tumour specific antibody or, possibly more effectively, immune complexes of antibody and tumour antigen. This may be effected simply by binding of tumour specific antibody (or immune complexes) to tumour cells so leading to a masking of the cell surface antigens. Interactions of this type may, however, lead to complex changes at the cell surface which result in a redistribution of tumour antigens or even to their loss by internalization or release (Nicolson, 1976). Whatever the specific reactions involved, the overall effect is that the cell surface associated tumour antigens will become unavailable for interaction with sensitized lymphoid cells, this being viewed as perhaps the most important component of the tumour rejection response.

Abrogation of cell mediated immunity in the tumour-bearing host may also be produced by tumour antigen and/or tumour specific immune complexes interacting directly with lymphoid cells so *inhibiting* their capacity to mediate cytotoxic reactions with tumour cells. This type of inhibitory response has been demonstrated with both experimental animal and human tumour systems by showing that the *in vitro* cytotoxicity of sensitized lymphoid cells, e.g. from tumour-free donors, can be abolished when they are exposed to tumour-bearer serum or isolated tumour antigen preparations (reviewed by Baldwin and Robins, 1975; Baldwin and Price, 1975). For example, the *in vitro* cytotoxicity of peripheral blood lymphocytes from colon carcinoma patients for cultured colon carcinoma cells can be inhibited by exposure of the effector cells to patient's serum (Nind *et al.*, 1975) or extracts containing the putative tumour antigen, isolated by papain digestion of tumour membrane fractions (Baldwin *et al.*, 1973). Using a similar approach, it has been shown that the reactivity of blood lymphocytes from patients with widely disseminated malignant melanoma is suppressed by a factor which can be eluted from melanoma cells, this also being present in patient's plasma (Currie and Basham, 1972).

Although the role of serum factors in the tumour-bearing host has not yet been adequately defined, it has been suggested that tumour antigen and/or immune complexes may be especially important because of their capacity to interfere with cell mediated immunity, but in addition tumour products may exert inhibitory effects in the local environment of the tumour. Whilst these hypotheses on the abrogation of tumour specific cell mediated immunity have been developed primarily to offer an explanation for the escape of nascent tumours from immunological control, they are also highly relevant in considering the immunobiology of metastatic spread of tumour cells. Tumour antigen containing factors released in the environment of the primary tumour may, for example, abrogate the effectiveness of local cell mediated immunity, thereby allowing tumour cells to escape into the circulation. It is also likely that the survival of circulating tumour cells will be enhanced if serum factors are present which specifically interfere with the cytotoxic capacity of sensitized lymphoid cells or if the tumour cells are blocked through the binding to tumour specific antibody.

1. Tumour antigen release and metastatic spread
The proposal that humoral factors modifying cell mediated immunity may be important in the metastatic process is supported by

studies (Currie and Alexander, 1974) showing that tumour antigen is rapidly shed from a metastasising rat sarcoma, Mc3, when cells were grown in tissue culture. In comparison, little tumour antigen was released in tissue culture medium from another rat sarcoma Mc1, and this particular tumour did not produce overt pulmonary metastases on subcutaneous implantation. From these comparative studies, it was suggested that pulmonary metastases from sarcoma Mc3 were able to develop, since tumour antigen released in the microenvironment of the primary tumour implant and secondary deposits effectively reduced the cell mediated response to tumour cell surface antigens. This is further supported by the finding that both sarcomas elicit cell mediated immunity against their tumour specific antigens, this being detected *in vitro* by the cytotoxicity of sensitized lymphocytes for cultured tumour cells. But only sarcoma Mc1 was capable of producing tumour rejection immunity and in this case rats pre-immunized against the tumour rejected a subsequent challenge with cells of the same tumour.

A similar correlation between metastatic potential and shedding of tumour cell surface components has been reported by Kim *et al.* (1975) from studies on a group of transplanted metastasising and non-metastasising rat mammary carcinomas. The three non-metastasising mammary carcinomas, originally induced with 3-methylcholanthrene, were immunogenic, immunoprotection being produced when normal rats were immunized with irradiated tumour cells. None of the metastasising mammary carcinomas were able to produce tumour rejection immunity when normal rats were immunized in a similar fashion with irradiated tumour cells. Electron microscopic studies of the surface characteristics of these tumours indicated that the metastasising mammary carcinomas had a thick glycocalyx, whereas the non-metastasising and immunogenic tumours had little or no glycocalyx. This, it was suggested, reflected the capacity of individual tumours to release plasma membrane components into the external environment.

IV. Immunotherapy of Metastatic Disease

A. *Non-specific Immunostimulation*

It is now well established that the growth of experimental animal tumours can sometimes be restricted by general host immunostimulation produced by systemic administration of bacterial adjuvants, particularly Bacillus Calmette Guérin BCG (reviewed by Laucius *et al.*, 1974; Bast *et al.*, 1974a, b, 1976) and, more recently, certain species of the anaerobic Corynebacteria, especially C. parvum (reviewed by Scott, 1974; Bast *et al.*, 1976). To completely prevent the growth of tumour transplants, systemic treatment by subcutaneous, intravenous or intraperitoneal injection, often has to be given several days before injection of tumour cells. While many tumours are retarded in their growth by this treatment, often a stimulation of growth is observed, and treatment can rarely affect growth of established disease.

In spite of the limitations of this treatment, a number of studies have been directed particularly to an evaluation of the influence of adjuvant-induced general immunostimulation on the growth of secondary tumour deposits (Table 3). For example, Sparks *et al.* (1974) working with a transplanted rat mammary carcinoma, have demonstrated that repeated subcutaneous injection of BCG after surgical removal of tumour grafts, prevented subsequent development of pulmonary metastases in about 50% of animals, compared with the dissemination of tumours in all animals receiving surgery alone. Bogden *et al.* (1974) working with the same tumour, investigated the effect of surgery, chemotherapy and immunotherapy alone and in combinations, and concluded that immunotherapy by systemic administration of soluble BCG extract, following chemotherapy and then surgical removal, was the most effective combination, all animals being cured of disease only by this combination therapy, with no recurrence or pulmonary, renal or hepatic metastases.

With Corynebacterium too, systemic administration can restrict the growth of disseminated tumour cells. Thus, subcutaneous administration of C. parvum restricts the growth of artificial pulmonary metastases produced from intravenously injected tumour cells (Bomford and Olivotto, 1974; Milas and Mujagic, 1972), although treatment was most effective if given up to 14 days before tumour injection. The related Corynebacterium, C. granulosum, similarly prevented development of pulmonary metastases from intravenously injected cells of murine sarcoma (Milas *et al.*, 1974b, c).

1. Clinical studies

Clinical trials have been initiated also to evaluate possible beneficial responses in patients receiving some form of immunostimulation therapy, in most instances this being introduced as an additional

TABLE 3

Immunostimulation for control of experimental metastases

Species	Tumour	Site of primary	Immunotherapy		Other treatment	Influence on metastases	Author
			Adjuvant	Route			
Rat	Mammary carcinoma	Subcutaneous	BCG	Subcutaneous	None	None	Sparks et al. (1974)
			BCG	Subcutaneous	Surgical removal of primary	Reduced hepatic and renal secondaries	
Rat	Mammary carcinoma	Subcutaneous	Methanol soluble fraction of BCG	Intraperitoneal	Chemotherapy, surgical removal of primary	Reduced hepatic and renal secondaries	Bogden et al. (1974)
Rat	Epithelioma	Subcutaneous	BCG	Intravenous	Surgical removal of primary	Reduced pulmonary secondaries	Baldwin and Pimm (1973a)
Mouse	Sarcoma	Cells injected intravenously	C. parvum	Subcutaneous, intraperitoneal or intravenous	None	Reduced pulmonary growth	Bomford and Olivotto (1974)
Mouse	Sarcoma	Cells injected intravenously	C. granulosum	Subcutaneous, intraperitoneal or intravenous	None	Reduced pulmonary growth	Milas et al. (1974b, c)
Mouse	Mammary carcinoma	Cells injected intravenously	C. granulosum	Subcutaneous, intraperitoneal or intravenous	None	Reduced pulmonary growth	Milas et al. (1974b)
Mouse	Sarcoma	Cells injected intravenously	C. parvum	Subcutaneous, intraperitoneal or intravenous	None	Reduced pulmonary growth	Milas and Mugagic (1972)

component to the conventional therapeutic approach. In general, this form of treatment is being evaluated in early malignancies or where there is minimal residual disease, since much of the experimental work suggests that host immune factors can only deal with a limited number of malignant cells (estimated to be of the order of 10^6 to 10^7 cells). This is not generally feasible, however, when considering the case of metastatic disease, so that in most of the current trials, immunological adjuvants are being introduced as an additional component, principally with combination chemotherapy (Table 4). In this respect, therefore, treatment with immunological adjuvants may not only enhance tumour-specific immune responses, but may also lead to repair of drug-induced damage to the host's immunological apparatus.

Almost all of the trials outlines in Table 4 are of recent origin, so that in most cases definitive clinical data are not yet available. Even so, conflicting findings are being presented which because of variables in the design of trials, e.g. type and dose of BCG used as well as methods of administration will be difficult to resolve. For example, one trial (Pinsky et al., 1976) was set up to determine

TABLE 4

Immunotherapy of metastatic cancer[a]

Disease	Therapy	Immunostimulation treatment	Author
Melanoma (Stages I and II)	Surgery ± DTIC	BCG Multiple puncture	Cunningham et al. (1977) Pinsky et al. (1976) Morton et al. (1976)
Melanoma (Disseminated)	MeCCNU	BCG scarification	Gutterman et al. (1975b)
Breast carcinoma (Disseminated)	5 FU, adriamycin, cyclophosphamide	BCG scarification	Gutterman et al. (1976b)
	Cyclophosphamide, adriamycin, methotrexate, 5 FU	C. parvum intradermal	Pinsky et al. (1977)
Colorectal carcinoma (Disseminated, Dukes C)	5 FU	BCG scarification	Gutterman et al. (1976c)
	5 FU, MeCCNU, (± vincristine)	MER intradermal	Moertal et al. (1975)
Lung carcinoma	Surgery Adriamycin	BCG intrapleural C. parvum subcutaneous	McKneally et al. (1976) Dimitrov et al. (1977)

See also International Conference on Immunotherapy of Cancer (*Ann. N. Y. Acad. Sci.* 227, 1–741, 1976).

whether BCG administration could prevent or delay recurrence in patients with malignant melanoma (Stage II) after removal of involved regional lymph nodes. Patients had to be "completely" free of disease to be eligible and therapy consisted of weekly adminis-tration of BCG (4 to 6 × 10⁷ viable units) by multiple puncture for 52 weeks followed by monthly injections. At two years the recurrence rate was 14/24 (58%) and 13/23 (57%) in the BCG treated and control groups. The median time to recurrence in the two groups was also similar and so it was concluded that in this study BCG administration was unable to prevent or delay recurrence of malignant melanoma. In comparison, two other malignant me-lanoma trials (Gutterman *et al.*, 1976a; Morton *et al.*, 1976) have reported increases in the disease-free interval from surgery as well as prolongation in survival in BCG treated patients. In other studies on patients with unresectable disseminated metastatic malignant me-lanoma (Stage IV), it has been reported that a beneficial response resulted from the inclusion of BCG together with dimethyl triazeno imidazole carboximide (DT1C) chemotherapy (Gutterman *et al.*, 1975a). The chemotherapy regimen was DT1C, 250 mg/m² in-travenously on days 1 to 5 of each treatment cycle. Fresh liquid Pasteur BCG, 6 × 10⁸ viable units, was given on days 7, 12 and 17 of each cycle and, where possible, courses were repeated every 12 days. Patients with clinical evidence of disseminated melanoma which was unresectable by surgery, were admitted to this trial. One report after a 32-month period indicated that 24/89 patients (27%) achieved a partial or complete remission and 28 additional patients (31%) had stabilization of the disease for greater than two months. Notably, patients with lymph node metastases (with or without subcutaneous metastases) had a remission rate of 55%. This was compared to a retrospective group of 104 consecutive patients treated with DT1C alone who had an overall remission rate of 18% in patients with lymph node metastases.

At this stage, it is not possible to provide unequivocal evaluation of the efficacy of BCG treatment in malignant melanoma, nor is the mechanism of action of BCG understood in any detail.

Objective regressions of metastases have also been reported in a small series of patients with metastatic gastrointestinal carcinoma following immunostimulation with the methanol extraction residue of BCG (Moertel *et al.*, 1975). The patients in this series all had far advanced cancer and either had failed to respond to chemotherapy or had shown progression after chemotherapy. MER was administered intradermally either at one week or at 4-week intervals and this led in a number of patients to an increase in immunological competence as assessed by a number of *in vivo* (e.g. response to recall antigens such as DNCB), or *in vitro* (e.g. mitogen-induced lymphocyte stimulation) assays. Of the 26 patients with measurable disease, 3 showed a greater than 50% regression of the most clearly measurable area of malignant disease which was chosen as the primary indicator lesion. For example in one patient, a 51-year-old woman with hepatic and peritoneal metastases, the lesions regressed completely 4 weeks after initiation of MER therapy. Both lesions were again demonstrable, however, by 12 to 15 weeks, together with pulmonary metastases but even though therapy was discontinued she was alive 11 months later. Interpretation of this type of trial is difficult, but the findings do provide at least an evaluation of the toxicity of the MER preparation for clinical trials in more suitable circumstances and, as pointed out by the authors, even the advanced cancer patients occasionally benefit.

Trials employing C. parvum to immunostimulate patients with disseminated cancer have also been reported (Israel *et al.*, 1975). In this series, twenty terminally ill patients with various disseminated tumours, including melanoma and lung and gastrointestinal carcinomas, were treated with daily intravenous infusions of C. parvum. Eight of the patients showed no response to therapy, four achieved a plateau in tumour progression, but in the other eight patients there was well-documented partial regression. For example, in one patient with carcinoma of the stomach, liver metastases underwent partial regression and this was maintained for 5 months with mitomycin C plus C. parvum treatment.

In these two recent investigations in advanced cancer patients, immunostimulation has been given to cases with an overwhelming tumour load primarily for the treatment of metastatic lesions. This would seem to contradict one line of thought, developed essentially from animal experimentation, that immunotherapy will be effective only against minimal residual disease. The objectives of these two approaches are, however, quite different, since it is hoped that immunotherapy of early, or minimum residual disease will be curative or at least result in significant regression of malignant disease. On the other hand, immunostimulation therapy of advanced cancer patients is only likely to prolong survival, so that its main objective would seem to be to increase the quality of life in terminal patients. Under these circumstances, therefore, treatment should be well tolerated, or at least be no more toxic than the alternative methods of patient management, e.g. cytostatic chemotherapy. This highlights the present dilemma in designing immunotherapy trials of disease, since many of the agents employed for immunostimulation, e.g. BCG, Corynebacterium parvum and MER have not been adequately evaluated in animal systems. Of particular importance in this respect is the toxicity of these substances when administered repeatedly over long periods of time, since in a number of clinical trials, toxic reactions to the therapy have been reported. This has already been documented in malignant melanoma treated by BCG, especially when the agent has been given intralesionally in patients with widely disseminated disease (Sparks et al., 1973) and there are also reports of toxic manifestations resulting from treatment with C. parvum (Band et al., 1975; Israel et al., 1975). From these comments it is far too premature to predict whether immune stimulation therapy will or will not contribute significantly to the treatment of malignant disease (reviewed by Mathé, 1976, and Mastrangelo et al., 1976). For example, it has been reported that BCG treatment added to chemotherapy prolongs remission and survival in patients with disseminated colorectal and breast cancer (Gutterman et al., 1976a). These studies remain to be confirmed, but even so it has to be recognized that repeated skin scarification with BCG may not be acceptable in patients with early disease.

B. *Adjuvant Contact Therapy*

Whilst bacterial adjuvants such as BCG and C. parvum may be introduced as general immunostimulants in the treatment of malignant disease, it has been established in experimental studies that infiltration of the adjuvants directly into the tumour site may often have a more marked effect on tumour growth. This form of treatment, referred to as adjuvent contact therapy, was originally demonstrated in tests on guinea-pig hepatomas, where it was shown that tumour cells injected in admixture with BCG did not produce palpable growth, and subsequently it was found that regression of tumours could be obtained following intralesional injection of BCG organisms (Zbar and Tanaka, 1971). Contact of BCG organisms has also been shown to suppress growth of other experimental transplanted tumours, including both carcinogen and virus-induced tumours as well as animal tumours arising without deliberate inducement, e.g. carcinogen-induced and spontaneous rat sarcomas and mammary carcinomas (Baldwin et al., 1976). To take an example, growth of cells derived from 3-methylcholanthrene-induced or spontaneous rat sarcomas injected into syngeneic rats can be completely prevented by the presence of BCG organisms. This is not produced by non-specific cytotoxic effects of the mycobacteria, since *in vitro* tumour cell killing cannot be demonstrated. Furthermore, the inhibition of tumour growth *in vivo* can be effected by a number of non-viable BCG preparations including radiation-attenuated whole organisms and subcellular fractions such as a methanol extraction residue (MER), and cell wall fragments on oil droplet emulsions (Baldwin *et al.*, 1974b; Hopper *et al.*, 1975; Baldwin and Pimm, 1973b).

Adjuvant contact suppression of tumour growth can also be effected with other microbial preparations including killed Crynebacterium parvum and Bordetella pertussis (Bast *et al.*, 1976) as well as double-stranded RNA isolated from a fungal virus (Pimm *et al.*, 1976). Corynebacterium parvum has been investigated in considerable detail for this purpose to assess its potential clinical application and several investigators have shown that tumour growth following transplantation of cells derived from a wide range of experimental tumours, e.g. mammary carcinomas, sarcomas and a melanoma in rats, mice and hamsters, can be suppressed by contacting the tumour cells with killed organisms (Paslin *et al.*, 1974; Likhite, 1974b; Woodruff and Dunbar, 1975).

The host responses involved in this type of adjuvant contact suppression are still far from being resolved, and are thought to include both lymphocyte and macrophage-mediated events. It is likely that the relative importance of the different cellular mechanisms will differ between different tumour types and between species. With BCG, however, there is a growing body of evidence that lymphocyte-mediated reactions are of lesser importance. This evidence is provided by studies showing that transplanted tumours can be suppressed by contacting with BCG even when the hosts are immunosuppressed by whole body irradiation (Moore *et al.*, 1975a, b; Pimm and Hopper, 1975; Pimm and Baldwin, 1976b). Furthermore, BCG-contact suppression of rat tumours can be obtained when tumours are implanted into congenitally athymic "nude" mice suggesting that T-lymphocyte mediated events are not necessarily required (Pimm and Baldwin, 1975a). Secondly, the site of adjuvant contact suppression shows histiocytic infiltration and granulomatous reactions suggesting the involvement of locally stimulated or activated macrophages (Hanna *et al.*, 1972). This idea is supported by the observations that, whilst rat tumour cells injected in admixture with BCG are inhibited from growth in normal animals, this effect can be abolished when the rats are pre-treated with silica preparations which act to specifically deplete host phagocytic cells

(Hopper *et al.*, 1976). Conversely, enrichment of tumour cell inocula with macrophages facilitates adjuvant contact suppression (Hopper and Pimm, 1976). Macrophages have been shown to be one of the major host cells normally invading experimental tumours (Evans, 1972; Van Loveren and Den Otter, 1974; Szymaniec and James, 1976; Baldwin, 1976a), and indeed there is a distinct correlation between the number of transplanted cells of a range of rat tumours which are suppressible by injection with BCG and the normal macrophage content of these inocula (Baldwin, 1976a). That is, tumours normally containing low macrophage contents (2%–10%) are less susceptible to adjuvant contact therapy with BCG than tumours with high macrophage infiltration (30%–40%).

Whatever the precise mechanisms involved in this adjuvant-induced host control of tumour growth, the technique of adjuvant contact therapy may have a particular application to the treatment of metastases. Firstly, intralesional injection of adjuvants may retard growth of the primary tumour and this may reduce metastatic spread. Alternatively, metastases developing at distant sites may be suppressed if adjuvants can be administered so that they reach the site of these secondary deposits.

1. Influence of adjuvant contact suppression of the primary tumour on metastatic spread

In tests with a transplanted rat osteosarcoma, originally induced with radioactive phosphorus, it was shown that growth of subcutaneous tumours was partially restricted by injection of tumour cells in admixture with BCG and the development of metastases in lung, liver and lymph nodes was restricted or in some cases completely prevented (Moore *et al.*, 1974, 1975a, b). In contrast, BCG injected at a site distant from the tumour inoculum exerted no influence either on the rate of subcutaneous tumour growth or on the secondary spread. Similar findings have been reported in studies with a transplanted rat epithelioma where injection of tumour cells in admixture with BCG not only retarded the appearance of sub-cutaneous tumours, but also markedly reduced the incidence of pulmonary metastases (Baldwin and Pimm, 1973a). In these studies with transplanted rat tumours, it was not established whether the reduction of metastases reflected only the retardation of growth of the initial tumour cell inoculum, or whether host responses initiated by the BCG component could specifically affect the rate of cell loss from the growing tumour, or influence their implantation elsewhere. Furthermore, attempts to modify metastatic spread by infiltrating established tumour grafts with BCG were not effective. Observations in other experimental tumour systems, such as the transplanted guinea-pig hepatoma, indicate however, that injection of BCG directly into established intradermal tumours caused local regression and, more importantly in the present context, prevented growth of metastases from tumour cells already seeded in the lymph nodes draining the site of tumour implantation so that about 60% of treated animals become tumour free (Zbar et al., 1972). In sharp contrast, surgical removal of intradermal tumours, while successfully effecting cures of the local growths, failed to influence the development of lymph node metastases which eventually proved fatal. Similarly, surgical resection of intradermal tumours and BCG injection at sites distant to the tumour was ineffective in suppressing lymph node metastases.

In the guinea-pig system described above, intralesional injection of BCG followed two days later by surgery was no more successful in effecting a total cure than simple intralesional injection of BCG. In tests with a rat mammary carcinoma it was also found that intralesional injection of BCG, followed 11 days later by surgical resection, was no more effective than surgery alone in preventing the subsequent appearance of lung, liver and kidney metastases (Sparks et al., 1974). In this particular system, however, in contrast to the guinea-pig hepatoma model, intralesional injections of BCG alone had little or no beneficial effect on growth of either the primary tumour or its metastases.

Other bacterial adjuvants too, have been shown to cause regression of localized tumours following intralesional injection and also to limit the growth of metastases, even if they were present in microscopic form at the time of treatment. For example, injections of C. granulosum into two-week-old established tumour grafts of a hamster melanoma caused their regression, animals remaining free of local tumour and of pulmonary metastases. In comparison, pulmonary metastases are generally present in hamsters with 2–3 week-old subcutaneous tumours and these developed progressively if the hamsters were not treated (Paslin et al., 1974). Similarly in tests with a rat mammary carcinoma, intralesionally administered C. parvum cured not only the local growth, but left all animals free of visceral and pulmonary metastases, even though these were present in 30%–60% of animals at the time of C. parvum injection (Likhite, 1974b). In contrast to the complete cure effected by C. parvum injection, 50% of animals undergoing surgical removal of the subcutaneous growth eventually died of metastases. Similar tests with killed

Bordetella pertussis demonstrated regression of intralesionally injected mouse mammary tumour transplants and prevention of
secondary deposits, although again the majority of mice undergoing
simple surgical removal died of widespread secondary deposits
(Likhite, 1974a).

2. Treatment of metastatic foci by direct adjuvant contact
As outlined above, a number of bacterial adjuvants when contacted
with tumour tissue can excite local host responses leading to tumour
suppression. This technique has a potential for treating metastatic
foci of malignant tissue if the adjuvant preparation can be administered
so that the material localizes at the site of metastases. Experimentally,
this type of treatment has been applied principally to the control of
pulmonary metastases, but deposits at other sites which are suitable
models for clinical situations are also susceptible to treatment.

(*a*) *Pulmonary metastases.* Studies with a range of transplanted rat
tumours demonstrated that, at least with 3-methylcholanthrene-
induced rat sarcomas, artificial pulmonary metastases, produced
from intravenously injected cells, could be eradicated by intravenous
injection of BCG organisms (Table 5), treatment being effective even
if given a few days after tumour cell injection (Baldwin and Pimm,
1973c). Under these circumstances, the tumour suppressive action is
probably a reflection of pulmonary entry of BCG organisms effecting
local stimulation of host responses, comparable to those produced
when cells and BCG are injected subcutaneously. This assumption is
supported by tests showing that up to 60% of radioactive labelled
BCG organisms will enter the lungs after intravenous injection,
indicating that close association between pulmonary micrometastases and the organism is possible, and histologically the lungs show a
haematogenous tuberculous reaction. Moreover, it should be noted
that BCG injected via any route other than intravenously, e.g. orally,
was not effective in controlling pulmonary tumour deposits (Baldwin
et al., 1975) although intrapleural injection of the vaccine is partially
effective (Pimm, 1976).

A number of similar studies have shown that intravenously
injected C. parvum can control growth of artificially produced
pulmonary metastases. In this case, however, it is not clear whether
tumour suppression resulted only from C. parvum infiltration of
tumour-containing pulmonary tissue, or from the very marked
general stimulation achieved with this agent. Thus, for example,
Bomford and Olivotto (1974) demonstrated protection against
intravenously injected mouse sarcoma cells by intravenously

TABLE 5

Adjuvant contact therapy of experimental metastases

Animal species	Primary tumour		Adjuvant treatment		Other treatment	Influence on metastases	Author
	Type	Site	Adjuvant	Route			
Rat	DBA-induced sarcoma	Footpad	BCG	Into popliteal lymph node	Surgical removal of primary	Reduced popliteal metastases	Carr and McGinty (1974)
Rat	Spontaneous epithelioma	Subcutaneous	BCG	Intravenous	Surgical removal of primary	Reduced pulmonary metastases	Baldwin and Pimm (1973a)
Rat	Primary DAB-induced hepatomas	Liver	BCG	Intravenous	None	Reduced pulmonary metastases	Baldwin and Pimm (1974)
Rat	MCA-induced sarcomas	Cells injected intravenously	BCG	Intravenous	None	Reduced pulmonary metastases	Baldwin and Pimm (1973c)
Rat	MCA-induced sarcomas	Cells injected intravenously	BCG	Intrapleurally	None	Reduced pulmonary metastases	Pimm (1976)
Guinea-pig	DENA-induced hepatoma	Intradermal	BCG	Into draining lymph node	Surgical removal of primary	Reduced lymph node metastases	Smith et al. (1975)
Guinea-pig	DENA-induced hepatoma	Intradermal	BCG	Into tumour	None	Reduced lymph node metastases	Zbar and Tanaka (1971)
Mouse	MCA-induced sarcoma	Cells injected intravenously	C. parvum	Intravenous	None	Reduced pulmonary metastases	Bomford and Olivotto (1974)

administered C. parvum. This effect was most marked when C. parvum was given 1–4 days before tumour cells, but C. parvum injected subcutaneously or intraperitoneally was equally effective.

In contrast to the results obtained with 3-methylcholanthrene-induced sarcomas, pulmonary growth from intravenously injected cells of other rat tumours including mammary carcinomas, an epithelioma and a sarcoma of spontaneous origin, was enhanced rather than suppressed following intravenous injection of BCG (Baldwin and Pimm, 1973c). The mechanisms involved in this enhancement are not yet clear, although it has been suggested that the effectiveness of BCG contact suppression may correlate with the macrophage content of developing tumours (see page 188) and tumours undergoing enhancement rather than suppression in the lung, generally show only a low degree of host macrophage infiltration (Baldwin, 1976a) and are only poorly suppressed by BCG even at the subcutaneous site. This type of finding does indicate, however, that the therapeutic effectiveness of new forms of treatment such as contacting bacterial adjuvants with metastatic deposits should be fully evaluated before clinical trial.

Based on the observations that at least some artificially formed pulmonary metastases could be suppressed by the introduction of BCG into lung tissue, further tests have indicated that intravenously injected BCG can control the development of spontaneous pulmonary metastases following surgical resection of the primary tumour. This has been established, for example, in tests with a transplanted rat epithelioma where the survival of animals from which subcutaneous growths had been excised was significantly prolonged and the incidence of pulmonary metastases reduced by post-operative intravenous administration of BCG (Baldwin and Pimm, 1973a). This therapeutic effect was most marked against pulmonary metastases, a number of animals being free of metastatic deposits at this site, but eventually succumbing with renal and dermal metastases. Following on from the experimental studies, clinical veterinary trials have been initiated to evaluate the effectiveness of this type of therapy in canine osteosarcoma (Owen; see Chapter V). In these cases, primary tumours were surgically resected and the dogs receiving additional intravenous BCG therapy showed prolongation of survival and restriction of pulmonary metastases.

In most experimental studies, the effect of adjuvant contact therapy on pulmonary metastases has been evaluated in animals rendered as tumour-free as possible, e.g. by surgical removal of local tumours. Tests with carcinogen-induced rat hepatomas, however, have shown that intravenously injected BCG can suppress both the incidence and extent of pulmonary metastases, even in the presence of progressively growing primary tumours (Baldwin and Pimm, 1974). In these experiments rats were fed for 90 days on a diet containing the hepatocarcinogen 4-dimethylaminoazobenzene, this constituting the period of carcinogen exposure when almost all animals can be expected to develop hepatocellular carcinomas. At this time, rats were transferred to a normal diet and treated with two intravenous injections of BCG seven and eleven days later. This resulted in fewer of the treated rats developing pulmonary metastases when compared with controls and even where metastases were formed there were fewer tumour foci. This effect was produced only against pulmonary metastases and is thought to result from BCG organisms localizing in lungs. However, treatment exerted no influence on the development of primary hepatic lesions.

(b) *Lymph node metastases.* With a transplanted carcinogen-induced sarcoma in the rat, Carr and McGinty (1974) found consistent lymph node metastases following footpad injection of tumour cells. The spread of tumour to draining popliteal nodes, could, however, be reduced by direct lymph node injection of BCG. Similarly, with a diethylnitrosamine-induced guinea-pig hepatoma, where the intralesional injection of BCG into intradermal tumours protected the animals against subsequent post-surgical lymph node metastases, intranodal injection of BCG at the time of graft excision also delayed the subsequent appearance of lymph node metastases and significantly prolonged survivals (Smith *et al.*, 1975).

(c) *Intraperitoneal and intrapleural tumours.* In addition to the treatment of pulmonary and lymph node metastases, infusion of adjuvants might be feasible as an adjunct to chemotherapy or surgery in the control of malignant effusions, particularly of the thorax These may occur, for example, from primary mesothelioma of the pleura, or may be secondary to carcinoma of lung or breast (*see* Martini *et al.*, 1975). This possibility has also been explored in studies with transplanted rat tumours where it has been shown that effusions and solid tumours in the pleural cavity can be controlled by intrapleurally administered BCG (Pimm and Baldwin, 1975b), Corynebacterium parvum (Pimm and Baldwin, 1976d) or double-stranded RNA (Pimm and Baldwin, 1976a). To take one example, rat sarcoma cells (10^6) injected intrapleurally rapidly form solid intrapleural growths so recipients have to be killed within fifteen days. These intrapleural growths can be completely arrested by intrapleural injection of BCG vaccine and in this experimental model, treatment (1×1 mg BCG Glaxo percutaneous vaccine) was effective when given on the day of tumour cell injection or up to 7 days later. Furthermore, a similar therapeutic response was obtained using radiation sterilized BCG vaccine as well as the methanol extraction residue (MER) of BCG. This is of considerable importance when considering the possible application of this type of infusion therapy in advanced cancer patients, where the development of mycobacterial infection from viable BCG organisms represents a real hazard and may require control by anti-tuberculous chemotherapy.

Experimental studies on the treatment of pulmonary metastases have emphasized the need for the adjuvant employed to localize in, or near to, the tumour site. Similarly, intrapleural tumours which are susceptible to intrapleural adjuvant therapy were not affected when BCG was administered by other routes, including intravenous, subcutaneous or intraperitoneal injection (Pimm and Baldwin, 1975b).

Intraperitoneal tumours have also been shown to be readily susceptible to adjuvants such as BCG and C. parvum when administered intraperitoneally, conditions which again allow tumour cell-adjuvant contact. For example, growth of rat sarcomas implanted intraperitoneally can be suppressed when BCG is also given by the intraperitoneal route, whereas BCG given by several other routes, e.g. subcutaneous or intravenous, has no effect (Pimm and Baldwin, 1975b).

3. Clinical studies

One of the problems inherent in any form of intralesional adjuvant therapy is to ensure that the agents employed are able to infiltrate the lesion. Furthermore, experimental evaluation indicates that this treatment is only likely to be effective with small tumour deposits, but, nevertheless adjuvant contact therapy may have potential value for treating small metastatic foci in man.

Clinically, the beneficial effects of intralesional adjuvant injection have been most definitely established in the treatment of patients with multiple dermal metastases from malignant melanoma. Originally Morton and his colleagues (Morton et al., 1970) reported that lesions injected with BCG frequently regressed and concomitantly, this could induce regression of other non-injected lesions. Morton et al. (1976) and many other investigators, principally Seigler et al. (1972), Nathanson (1972), Bornstein et al. (1973) and Pinsky et al. (1973) have confirmed and extended these observations and Bast et al. (1974b) in reviewing the application of BCG for the treatment of human cancer have collected reports on 12 groups using this form of treatment for dermal malignant melanoma. Overall, lesions injected with BCG regressed in 58% of cases, but the effect on non-injected lesions was not so impressive, a regression rate of only 14% being observed.

However, two important factors correlate with the success of this type of BCG treatment (Morton et al., 1976). Firstly, generally good immunocompetence, as judged by delayed cutaneous hypersensitivity reactions to materials such as DNCB (dinitrochlorobenzene) or conversion to DNCB reactivity following BCG treatment, generally resulted in a good response to intralesional BCG injections. Secondly, patients with subcutaneous, rather than dermal metastases generally have a poor response, and while some injected lesions may regress there is rarely a concomitant regression of uninjected lesions. The effect of intralesional injection of BCG into dermal melanoma metastases also produces a poor response in visceral metastases, but this situation has so far not been adequately resolved. For example, there is one report of a patient where injection of intracutaneous melanoma metastases with BCG resulted in an objective regression of pulmonary metastatic disease (Mastrangelo et al., 1975).

Intralesional BCG injection has also been attempted in seven patients with adenocarcinoma of the prostate where hormonal therapy had failed (Merrin et al., 1975). Five patients had a decrease in the size and induration of the prostate and in one, the treatment produced tumour necrosis. No changes were observed, however, in measurable metastases except in one patient where a soft tissue lesion injected directly with BCG showed necrosis and the general condition in four of the seven patients worsened.

In addition to the treatment of solid secondary deposits, adjuvant contact therapy is also being evaluated for effectiveness against malignant effusions secondary to mammary carcinoma or developing from primary mesothelioma of the pleura. In the case of mesothelioma, patients with relatively advanced disease, and receiving no other treatment, repeated intrapleural administration of increasing doses of radiation killed BCG can lead to a reduction in the rate of accumulation of pleural fluid (Elmes, 1976). Similarly, patients with pleural effusions secondary to mammary carcinoma, in whom effusions were not responsive to conventional therapy, may show beneficial responses to intrapleurally administered BCG (Pimm and Baldwin, 1976c).

In the treatment of lung cancer too, McKneally et al. (1976) have demonstrated beneficial effects and prolongation of survival in patients receiving a single post-operative injection of BCG into the pleural space after surgery for Stage I disease. It is not clear in this instance, however, whether this effect really depends upon regional application of the vaccine, since beneficial effects have also been observed in lung cancer following BCG injection at distant, intradermal sites (Edwards and Whitewell, 1974; Pines, 1976).

Clearly there is a problem in the extension of this type of therapy to secondary deposits not so readily accessible to infiltration with adjuvants as cutaneous or pleural sites. Experimental studies, reviewed in Section 2, indicate that more disseminated disease, particularly pulmonary metastases might be controlled by a systemic, intravenous administration of adjuvant. Clinically, such treatment has to be approached with great caution, but, nevertheless, toxicological studies with BCG injected intravenously into primates, including man, indicate that such a procedure is feasible. In man, Schwarzenberg et al. (1976) have injected a small group of cancer patients with melanoma or leukaemia with live BCG vaccine and observed chills, high fever and vomiting in the majority, with hepatic granuloma formation. This mode of administration did not induce any restoration in immunosuppressed patients, and indeed produced immunosuppression in 3/4 patients allergic to skin test antigens. The production of immunosuppression by large doses of intravenously injected vaccine has been described experimentally in mice by Geffard and Orbach-Arbouys (1976) and further emphasizes the need for added caution in clinical injection of the vaccine by this route. In baboons, Jurczyk-Procyk et al. (1976) have demonstrated cellular infiltration of macrophages and lymphocytes in liver, lung, spleen and lymph nodes, with granuloma formation in liver, lungs and spleen, in animals injected intravenously with viable BCG. After four to five months, granulomas regressed, but viable organisms were still demonstrable in lymph nodes. This type of persistent infection might be avoided if killed BCG organisms replaced viable vaccine, and for adjuvant contact therapy, BCG killed by γ-irradiation is as effective as living vaccine in experimental systems (Baldwin et al., 1974b) although it still produces liver and lung granulomas in tuberculin sensitive animals (Muggleton et al., 1975).

The possibility of systemic administration of Corynebacterium parvum too, has been indicated by Israel et al. (1975), who have repeatedly injected killed C. parvum organisms intravenously into twenty patients, terminally ill with various disseminated tumours. Partial regression of lesions to less than half their original size was seen in 8 (40%) of patients. These authors concluded that intravenously injected C. parvum was without serious toxicity, although chills and high fever, similar to those observed following intravenous BCG administration, were seen in all patients. In contrast to the effect of

BCG, however, skin test hypersensitivity reactions to DNCB did not change following C. parvum administration, the only patient who converted from negative to positive showing no clinical response to treatment.

A similar study by Band *et al.* (1975) has also indicated the possibility of intravenous C. parvum injection to treat patients with a variety of tumour types. Major toxic effects included rigors and cyanosis, hypertension, nausea and vomiting but toxicity decreased on repeated administration of the vaccine. Objective tumour regression occurred in 4/19 patients, the most marked of which was a patient with multiple pulmonary metastases from osteogenic sarcoma, in whom all but one pulmonary lesion underwent regression following intravenous C. parvum treatment.

These preliminary results with both BCG and C. parvum are encouraging and warrant further investigation. However, the necessity for extensive experimental evaluation of the immunological effects of such treatment in normal and tumour-bearing animals cannot be stressed too strongly.

C. *Active Immunotherapy*

It has been conclusively established in many experimental tumour systems that pre-immunization, e.g. by implantation of radiation-attenuated tumour cells, can provide the host with a moderate degree of protection against a subsequent challenge with cells of the immunizing tumour. In many cases, it has also been found that this tumour immune rejection response can be enhanced by incorporating immunological adjuvants such as BCG in the treatment protocol, often in the form of mixed tumour cell-adjuvant vaccine. For example, little or no host resistance to tumour challenge could be demonstrated in guinea-pigs following surgical resection of a transplanted hepatoma, whereas animals treated with a vaccine containing irradiated tumour cells and BCG were immune (Bartlett and Zbar, 1972).

The finding of immunity in animals rejecting vaccines containing tumour cells and adjuvants, has led several investigators to explore the feasibility of using mixed inocula for specific active immunotherapy of primary tumours as well as metastatic deposits. For example, with a guinea-pig hepatoma model, animals were challenged subcutaneously on one side of the body and treated at a contralateral site with tumour cells admixed with BCG. This treatment resulted in suppression of growth at the challenge site after a transient development of tumour; under the optimum conditions palpable established growths (up to

15 mm diameter) being rejected completely due to the development of a systemic tumour-specific immunity (Bartlett and Zbar, 1972). Either viable or irradiated (12,000 R) tumour cells could be used for this form of immunotherapy, although vaccines containing viable cells occasionally produced progressively growing tumours. This illustrates one of the dilemmas in designing suitable vaccines for active immunotherapy, since in many experimental studies vaccines containing adjuvant mixed with viable tumour cells are more effective than those containing inactivated tumour cells, e.g. following irradiation or cytotoxic drug treatment. For example, studies with transplanted rat sarcomas showed that subcutaneous tumour challenges were most effectively controlled by contralateral treatment with viable sarcoma cells mixed with BCG, while vaccines containing γ-irradiated (15,000 R) or mitomycin C-treated cells were only partially effective (Baldwin and Pimm, 1973b). In comparison, however, treatment of mice with irradiated tumour cells mixed with C. parvum and injected into the footpad effectively controlled growth of subcutaneously injected cells from a chemically-induced sarcoma (Bomford, 1975).

It should be emphasized that active immunotherapy with tumour cells, whether with or without the incorporation of immunological adjuvants into the vaccine, is mediated by specific tumour immune responses evoked against tumour associated rejection antigens. For example, it is well known that the major class of tumour rejection antigen associated with animal tumours induced by chemical carcinogens are highly specific components on individual tumours (Baldwin, 1973). In accord with this, treatment of guinea-pigs with vaccines containing BCG admixed with cells of one hepatoma (Line 10) controlled growth of this tumour at a contralateral site, whereas treatment was ineffective against another immunologically distinct hepatoma (Line 1) (Bartlett and Zbar, 1972). Furthermore, generation of a tumour specific immune response in tumour-bearing animals treated by vaccines containing tumour cells with immunological adjuvants is dependent upon the host having adequate immunocompetence. For example, the therapeutic effect observed against a transplanted mouse sarcoma following contralateral treatment with irradiated tumour cells mixed with C. parvum was abrogated when the hosts were depleted of T cells by neonatal thymectomy and whole body irradiation (Bomford, 1975). Furthermore, even less severe forms of immunosuppression (450 R whole body irradiation) was found to abolish the capacity of rat sarcoma cells admixed with BCG to suppress growth of a contralateral challenge with cells of the same tumour (Pimm and Hopper, 1975; Pimm and Baldwin, 1976b) so that this form of therapy is likely to be less effective if attempted in hosts with diminished immunocompetence.

Even with the above limitations, there is evidence indicating that active immunotherapy can be employed in the treatment of metastatic deposits. One experimental model now being used for evaluating this involves treatment of "artificial" pulmonary metastases produced following intravenous injection of tumour cells. For example, pulmonary growth of intravenously transferred rat sarcoma cells was partially suppressed by a single or repeated subcutaneous injection of a vaccine containing viable tumour cells together with BCG (Baldwin and Pimm, 1973c) Vaccines containing irradiated tumour cells admixed with C. parvum have also been employed for the treatment of artificial pulmonary metastases produced following intravenous injection of murine sarcoma cells (Milas et al., 1975). In both these studies, active immunotherapy resulted in a reduction of the numbers of pulmonary tumour nodules developing, but did not completely eradicate pulmonary disease, so that all of the animals eventually had to be killed. Under these conditions, therefore, the response to active immunotherapy was much less effective than that achieved by allowing intravenously injected adjuvants to contact with tumour cell deposits, since this often resulted in total suppression of pulmonary tumour deposits (Baldwin and Pimm, 1973c). A similar conclusion was drawn from studies with a transplanted rat epithelioma which produces pulmonary metastases when implanted subcutaneously (Baldwin and Pimm, 1973a). In these tests, where local subcutaneous tumour was surgically resected and attempts made to treat pulmonary metastases, active immunotherapy employing an irradiated tumour cell-BCG vaccine was ineffective. Some measure of control of pulmonary metastases was achieved following intravenous injection of BCG, but this response was not enhanced by simultaneous attempts to boost specific tumour immunity employing an irradiated tumour cell-BCG vaccine.

1. Clinical studies

The clinical potential of active immunotherapy still remains to be evaluated, although encouraging results have been reported, particularly in the treatment of haematological malignancies. The earlier trials of Mathé (Mathé et al., 1969, 1973, 1976) on the immunotherapy of acute lymphocytic leukaemia, where one of the therapeutic components was active immunization with irradiated allogeneic leukaemic cells, are now well known. In these trials, attempts were made to take into account findings from studies with experimental murine leukaemias that only small numbers of tumour cells (10^5 to 10^6) could be rejected by active immunization. Accordingly, treatment was initiated in conjunction with so-called "cytoreductive chemotherapy", the objective being to bring the tumour cell population down to a level that, it was predicted, could be dealt with by host immune responses. Several trials have also been introduced for the treatment of acute myeloblastic leukaemia, where patients received immunization with irradiated allogeneic leukaemia cells, together with BCG either incorporated into the vaccine or injected into different sites (reviewed by Powles, 1976). Again, these studies have produced encouraging results in terms of prolongation of remission in patients receiving immunotherapy plus chemotherapy compared to chemotherapy alone. However, the trials are still of insufficient duration to allow conclusive validation of the concept of active immunotherapy.

In addition to the treatment of leukaemias there are a number of trials where active immunization, generally with attenuated tumour cells and often in combination with an adjuvant such as BCG, are being carried to evaluate this type of treatment in the control of metastatic disease from solid tumours. Most of these trials have only been carried out for a short time so that information is not yet available on their effectiveness. There are, however, a number of fundamental problems still to be resolved before treatment of metastatic disease can be logically designed. Basically this depends upon whether the concept developed from experimental animal studies, that the host's immune system is only able to reject modest amounts of tumour is accepted. If so, this implies that active immunotherapy will be applicable only for the treatment of microscopic metastatic deposits. Introduction of this form of treatment, therefore, may be dependent upon the introduction of more sensitive methods of detecting residual tumour deposits.

D. *Immunotherapy by Passively Transferred Effector Cells and Humoral Factors*

As discussed in the Introduction, passive transfer of lymphocytes or macrophages to syngeneic recipient animals may transfer tumour immunity from sensitized donors. Serum from immune donors is generally less effective at transferring immunity, and may enhance, rather than suppress, tumour growth in recipient animals, probably because of serum-borne enhancing antibodies. A number of recent studies have indicated the possibility of controlling the growth of secondary deposits of tumour with passively transferred lymphocytes or stimulated macrophages or serum-borne factors, although these later may be factors capable of stimulating anti-tumour activity of recipient tumour host macrophages rather than simple antibodies.

1. Sensitized lymphocytes and macrophages
Fidler (1974a) in tests with the transplanted B16 mouse melanoma demonstrated that the intravenous injection of tumour cells together with lymphocytes from B16-immune mice in a ratio of 5000:1, dramatically reduced the incidence of pulmonary tumour growths initiated by the intravenous injection of tumour cells, compared with the effect of normal, tumour bearer or non-specifically sensitized lymphocytes. However, a lower ratio of lymphocytes to tumour cells enhanced rather than suppressed pulmonary tumour growth, but this effect was observed with normal lymphocytes too, and could be ascribed to increased pulmonary trapping of tumour cell lymphocyte clumps produced during *in vitro* inoculation prior to injection. The feasibility of using passively transferred lymphocytes to treat established pulmonary deposits was not examined. However in further studies with the mouse melanoma B16, Fidler (1974b) has also demonstrated a therapeutic effect of intravenously transferred acti vated macrophages against established pulmonary growths of tumour. It is known that immunologically sensitized lymphocytes on contact with the immunizing antigen may release a number of biologically active materials, some of which are chemotactic to macrophages and may activate them to a state cytotoxic for malignant cells (reviewed by David, 1971). In experiments to assess the therapeutic effect of such activated macrophages against secondary tumour deposits, macrophages from mice bearing subcutaneous melanoma growths were treated *in vitro* with supernatants from cultured B16 melanoma cells alone or tumour cells and xenogeneic (rat) lymphocytes from normal rats, non-specifically immune rats or rats immunized against the B16 mouse melanoma. Inhibition of mouse pulmonary tumour growths, initiated two days before by the intravenous injection of cells, was achieved with intravenously administered macrophages exposed to supernatants from B16 cells and specifically sensitized rat lymphocytes. Supernatants from mixtures of lymphocytes from rats immunized with a different tumour and B16 cells were only partially effective, and culture supernatants of B16 cells alone or B16 cells and normal lymphocytes were inactive. It is probable that the antitumour effect of the activated macrophages against pulmonary tumour growths was effected by these cells after lodgment in the lungs after intravenous injection, although no definitive demonstration of these

mechanisms was attempted. Nevertheless, the indication is that such macrophages might be effective in controlling secondary deposits at other sites if directed towards these metastases.

2. Serum borne factors

Clearly macrophages in tumour bearing animals with the B16 melanoma described above are either not activated by cytotoxicity against malignant tissue or they are not sufficiently effective, since progressive growth of primary and metastatic deposits usually occurs. However, studies by Proctor et al. (1973) with chemically-induced rat sarcomas have demonstrated the presence of a circulating humoral factor, putatively not an antibody, specifically capable of controlling the growth of secondary tumour deposits, possibly by its in vivo activation of macrophages. With transplanted tumours which rarely metastasised from intramuscular growths, prolonged drainage of thoracic duct lymph encouraged dissemination to the lungs. Return of drained lymphocytes failed to prevent this encouragement of meta-stasis, suggesting that removal of a humoral rather than a cellular factor was permitting tumour dissemination. In tests on the therapy of artificial pulmonary metastases produced by the intravenous injection of cells, passive transfer of tumour-bearer serum suppressed tumour growth. This effect was specifically directed against secondary deposits of the tumour borne intramuscularly by the serum donor. No therapeutic effect could be achieved against localized intramuscular deposits, only against disseminated tumour. It was thought unlikely that the serum factor involved was conventional antibody, because such sera contained no free antibody demonstrable by immunofluores-cence or mixed cell agglutination reactions.

3. Removal of circulating blocking factors

As discussed previously, the failure of cell mediated immune responses to control the growth of primary or secondary tumour deposits may be due, at least in part, to the presence in tumour bearing animals of circulating serum factors (antigen-antibody complexes) capable of abrogating the expression of lymphocyte cytotoxicity against tumour cells. The removal of these blocking substances might, therefore, permit more effective host control of primary or disseminating tumour. For example, removal of the spleen has been reported to decrease humoral antibody responses to experimental tumours and inhibit their local development (Ferrer and Mihich, 1968; Pollack, 1971), and also to suppress the development of pulmonary metastases resulting from intravenous injection of tumour cells (Milas and

Mujagic, 1973). In addition, *in vitro* studies (Hellström and Hellström, 1970; Bansal and Sjögren, 1971; Robins and Baldwin, 1974) have demonstrated that certain syngeneic or xenogeneic anti-tumour antisera can prevent the blocking activity of tumour-bearer sera for cytotoxic lymphocytes suggesting the possible use of such sera in *in vivo* "unblocking". In this context, in a series of tests with polyoma virus induced tumours in rats, Bansal and Sjögren (1973) have demonstrated that the treatment of animals with these unblocking antisera can reduce the levels of circulating blocking factors and beneficially influence the growth of secondary tumour deposits. Rats from which progressively growing subcutaneous polyoma tumours were surgically excised, were given a second injection of cells at a distant site, splenectomized (to reduce further antibody production) and treated by repeated intraperitoneal injections of unblocking syngeneic antisera. The treatment resulted in subsequent regression of the secondary deposit in a total of 12/23 rats. A disappearance of serum blocking was seen in all rats with regressing tumours, but in animals in which treatment was unsuccessful high levels of blocking activity were maintained. The unblocking serum used in these tests was obtained from BCG primed syngeneic rats a few days after the subcutaneous injection of polyoma tumour cells, but other studies (Bansal and Sjögren, 1971) indicate the feasibility of using xenogeneic antisera prepared similarly in rabbits. In further tests with transplanted polyoma tumours an attempt was made to treat spontaneous metastases appearing after surgical removal of large subcutaneous tumour deposits. Here treatment with unblocking antisera prolonged survivals of animals and this was associated with reduced dissemination of the tumour.

V. Conclusions

There is now conclusive evidence from studies with experimental animal tumours that host recognition of tumour associated antigens may lead to the development of tumour rejection responses which can influence growth of the primary lesion as well as metastatic deposits. It is also evident from experimental immunotherapy research that tumour immunity can be enhanced in a number of ways which may have therapeutic value. In this connection however, it must be recognized that current knowledge of the highly complex immune responses developing in the tumour bearing host as distinct from the pre-immunized normal animal are still only poorly understood

(Baldwin and Robins, 1977). It is possible, therefore, that more effective methods of stimulating tumour immunity may be developed in the future. This is especially pertinent in considering immunotherapeutic protocols, since many of the reagents currently employed, e.g. BCG and C. parvum are likely to prove unsuitable for long-term administration. Hopeful research into the mechanism of action of these bacterial products will lead to the development of more well-defined therapeutically active substances, preferably without undesirable toxic side effects.

Perhaps the most important problem arising to some extent from the rapid expansion of work in the field of tumour immunology, is the general acceptance that all human tumours will have tumour associated antigens against which the host is able to mount tumour rejection responses (Baldwin, 1976b). It has already been established that this is not so with some animal tumours, notably those arising naturally (Baldwin and Embleton, 1974; Klein and Klein, 1977) and this constitutes an important challenge in human tumour immunology. Unfortunately, at the present many of the *in vitro* techniques introduced for detecting human tumour antigens are viewed as being unsatisfactory (Baldwin and Embleton, 1977), and so there is a dilemma in introducing immunotherapy for the treatment of human malignant disease. Undoubtedly immunotherapy trials will continue and many of them will be introduced under conditions where the existing knowledge from experimental tumour studies would indicate little chance of success. This is especially relevant to the treatment of disseminated tumour, since in most experimental studies only limited numbers of tumour cells can be suppressed by immune mechanisms. These basic problems in the conduct of immunotherapy trials for both local and metastatic disease need to be recognized so that the limited success which may accrue from current trials is not received too pessimistically. In this context it is necessary to recognize that immunotherapy is in its "infancy" and the lessons of slow progress over the past 25 years in chemotherapy research need to be accepted.

Acknowledgement

The authors' work was supported by a departmental grant from the Cancer Research Campaign.

References

Alexander, P., Bensted, J., Delorme, E. J., Hall, J. G. and Hodgett, J. (1969). *Proc. Roy. Soc. Lond. B.* **174**, 237–251.
Baldwin, R. W. (1973). *Advan. Cancer Res.* **18**, 1–75.
Baldwin, R. W. (1975). *J. Natl. Cancer Inst.* **55**, 745–748.
Baldwin, R. W. (1976a). *Transplant. Rev.* **28**, 62–74.
Baldwin, R. W. (1976b). *Cancer Immunol. Immunother.* **1**, 197–198.
Baldwin, R. W. and Embleton, M. J. (1974). *Int. J. Cancer*, **13**, 433–443.
Baldwin, R. W. and Embleton, M. J. (1977). *Int. Rev. Exptl. Path.* **17**, 49–95.
Baldwin, R. W. and Pimm, M. V. (1973a). *Int. J. Cancer*, **12**, 420–427.
Baldwin, R. W. and Pimm, M. V. (1973b). *Nat. Cancer Inst. Monogr.* **39**, 11–17.
Baldwin, R. W. and Pimm, M. V. (1973c). *Brit. J. Cancer*, **27**, 48–54.
Baldwin, R. W. and Pimm, M. V. (1974). *Brit. J. Cancer*, **30**, 473–476.
Baldwin, R. W. and Price, M. R. (1975). *In* "Cancer: A Comprehensive Treatise" (F. F. Becker, ed.), Vol. 1, pp. 353–383. Plenum Press, New York.
Baldwin, R. W. and Robins, R. A. (1975). *Curr. Top. Microbiol. Immunol.* **72**, 21–53.
Baldwin, R. W. and Robins, R. A. (1976). *Brit. Med. Bull.* **32**, 118–123.
Baldwin, R. W. and Robins, R. A. (1977). *In* "Contemporary Topics in Molecular Immunology" (G. L. Ada and R. R. Porter, eds), Vol. 6, pp. 177–207. Plenum Press, New York.
Baldwin, R. W., Embleton, M. J. and Price, M. R. (1973). *Int. J. Cancer*, **12**, 84–92.
Baldwin, R. W., Embleton, M. J., Price, M. R. and Vose, B. M. (1974a). *Transplant. Rev.* **20**, 77–99.
Baldwin, R. W., Cook, A. J., Hopper, D. G. and Pimm, M. V. (1974b). *Int. J. Cancer*, **13**, 743–750.
Baldwin, R. W., Hopper, D. G. and Pimm, M. V. (1975). *Brit. J. Cancer*, **31**, 124–128.
Baldwin, R. W., Hopper, D. G. and Pimm, M. V. (1976) *Ann. N. Y. Acad. Sci.* **277**, 124–134.
Band, P. R., Jao-King, C., Urtasun, R. C. and Haraphongse, M. (1975). *Cancer Chemotherapy Reps.* **59**, 1139–1145.
Bansal, S. C. and Sjögren, H. O. (1971). *Nature, Lond., New Biol.* **233**, 76–78.
Bansal, S. C. and Sjögren, H. O. (1973). *Int. J. Cancer*, **12**, 179–193.
Bartlett, G. L. (1972). *J. Natl. Cancer Inst.* **49**, 493–504.
Bartlett, G. L. and Zbar, B. (1972). *J. Natl. Cancer Inst.* **48**, 1709–1726.
Bast, R. C., Zbar, B., Borsos, T. and Rapp, H. J. (1974a). *New Engl. J. Med.* **290**, 1413–1420.
Bast, R. C., Zbar, B., Borsos, T. and Rapp, H. J. (1974b). *New Engl. J. Med.* **290**, 1458–1469.
Bast, R. C., Bast, B. S. and Rapp, H. J. (1976). *Ann. N. Y. Acad. Sci.* **277**, 60–92.
Bogden, A. E., Esber, H. J., Taylor, D. J. and Gray, J. H. (1974). *Cancer Res.* **34**, 1627–1631.
Bomford, R. (1975). *Brit. J. Cancer*, **32**, 551–558.
Bomford, R. and Olivotto, M. (1974). *Int. J. Cancer*, **14**, 226–235.
Bornstein, R. S., Mastrangelo, M. J., Sulit, H., Chee, D., Yarbro, J. W., Prehn, L. M. and Prehn, R. T. (1973). *Nat. Cancer Inst. Monogr.* **39**, 213–220.
Carnaud, C., Hoch, B. and Trainin, N. (1974). *J. Natl. Cancer Inst.* **52**, 395–399.
Carr, I. and McGinty, F. (1974). *J. Path.* **113**, 85–95.
Chandradasa, K. D. (1973). *Int. J. Cancer*, **11**, 648–662.
Cikes, M. and Klein, G. (1972). *J. Natl. Cancer Inst.* **48**, 509–515.

Crile, G. (1968). *Surgery, Gynaecology, Obstetrics*, **126**, 1270–1272.

Cunningham, T. J., Schoenfeld, D., Walters, J., Nathanson, L., Cohen, M. and Paterson, B. (1977). *In* "Immunotherapy of Cancer: Present Status of Trials in Man". Raven Press, New York. In press.

Currie, G. A. and Alexander, P. (1974). *Brit. J. Cancer*, **29**, 72–75.

Currie, G. A. and Basham, C. (1972). *Brit. J. Cancer*, **26**, 427–438.

David, J. R. (1971). *In* "Progress in Immunology" (D. B. Amos, ed.), Vol. 1, pp. 399–412. Academic Press, New York and London.

Deckers, P. J., Davis, R. C., Parker, G. A. and Mannick, J. A. (1973). *Cancer Res.* **33**, 33–39.

Deichman, G. I. and Kluchareva, T. E. (1966). *J. Natl. Cancer Inst.* **36**, 647–655.

Deodhar, S. D. and Crile, G. (1969). *Cancer Res.* **29**, 776–779.

Dimitrov, N. Y., Conroy, J., Suhrland, L. G., Singh, T. and Teitlebaum, H. (1977). *In* "Immunotherapy of Cancer: Present Status of Trials in Man". Raven Press, New York. In press.

Eccles, S. A. and Alexander, P. (1974). *Nature, Lond.* **250**, 667–669.

Eccles, S. A. and Alexander, P. (1975). *Nature, Lond.* **257**, 52–53.

Edwards, F. R. and Whitewell, F. (1974). *Thorax*, **29**, 654–665.

Elmes, P. C. (1976). Personal communication.

Evans, R. (1972). *Transplantation*, **14**, 468–473.

Faraci, R. P. (1974). *Surgery*, **76**, 469–473.

Ferrer, J. F. and Mihich, E. (1968). *Cancer Res.* **28**, 1116–1120.

Fidler, I. J. (1974a). *Cancer Res.* **34**, 491–498.

Fidler, I. J. (1974b). *Cancer Res.* **34**, 1074–1078.

Fisher, B., Soliman, O. and Fisher, E. R. (1969a). *Proc. Soc. Exp. Biol. Med. (N.Y.)* **131**, 16–18.

Fisher, E. R., Soliman, O. and Fisher, B. (1969b). *Nature, Lond.* **221**, 287–288.

Fisher, B., Saffers, E. A. and Fisher, E. R. (1970). *Proc. Soc. Exp. Biol. Med.* **135**, 68–71.

Flannery, G. R., Chalmers, P. J., Rolland, J. M. and Nairn, R. C. (1973). *Brit. J. Cancer*, **28**, 118–122.

Forman, J. and Möller, G. (1973). *Transplant. Rev.* **17**, 108–149.

Geffard, M. and Orbach-Arbuoys, S. (1976). *Cancer Immunol. Immunother.* **1**, 41–43.

Gershon, R. K. and Carter, R. L. (1970). *Nature, Lond.* **226**, 368–370.

Gershon, R. K., Carter, R. L. and Kondo, K. (1967). *Nature, Lond.* **213**, 674–676.

Gershon, R. K., Carter, R. L. and Kondo, K. (1968). *Science*, **159**, 646–648.

Goldman, L. I., Flaxman, B. A. Wernick, G. and Zabriskie, J. B. (1974). *Surgery*, **76**, 50–56.

Gutterman, J. U., Mavligit, G., Gottlieb, J., Burgess, M. A., McBride, C. E., Einhorn, L., Freireich, E. J. and Hersh, E. M. (1975a). *Behring Inst. Mitt.* **56**, 235–250.

Gutterman, J. U., Mavligit, G. M., Reed, R. C., Burgess, M. A., McBride, C. M. and Hersh, E. M. (1975b). *Behring Inst. Mitt.* **56**, 199–206.

Gutterman, J. U., Mavligit, G. M., Burgess, M. A., Cardenas, J. O., Blumenschein, G. R., Gottlieb, J. A., McBride, C. M., McCredie, K. B., Bodey, G. P., Rodriguel, V., Freireich, E. J. and Hersh, E. M. (1976a). *Cancer Immunol. Immunother.* **1**, 99–107.

Gutterman, J. U., Blumenschein, G. R., Hortobagyi, G., Mavligit, G. and Hersh, E. M. (1976b). *Breast, Diseases of the Breast*, **2**, 29–34.

Gutterman, J. V., Mavligit, G. M., Blumenshein, G., Burgess, M. A., McBride, C. M. and Hersh, E. M. (1976c). *Ann. N. Y. Acad. Sci.* **277**, 135–158.
Hammond, W. G., Rolley, R. T. and Sparks, F. C. (1968). *Proc. Am. Assoc. Cancer Res.* **9**, 27.
Hanna, M. G., Jr., Zbar, B. and Rapp, H. J. (1972) *J. Natl. Cancer Inst.* **48**, 1441–1455.
Hellström, I. and Hellström, K. E. (1969). *Int. J. Cancer*, **4**, 587–600.
Hellström, I. and Hellström, K. E. (1970). *Int. J. Cancer*, **5**, 195–201.
Hellström, K. E. and Hellström, I. (1974). *Advan. Immunol.* **18**, 209–277.
Hellström, I., Hellström, K. E. and Sjögren, H. O. (1970). *Cell Immunol.* **1**, 18–30.
Herberman, R. B. (1976). *In* "Mechanisms of Tumor Immunity" (I. Green, S. Cohen, R. T. McCluskey, eds). J. Wiley & Sons, Inc., New York.
Herberman, R. B. and Oldham, R. K. (1975). *J. Natl. Cancer Inst.* **55**, 749–753.
Hopper, D. G. and Pimm, M. V. (1976). *Lancet*, **2**, 255–256.
Hopper, D. G., Pimm, M. V. and Baldwin, R. W. (1975). *Brit. J. Cancer*, **31**, 176–181.
Hopper, D. G., Pimm, M. V. and Baldwin, R. W. (1976). *Cancer Immunol. Immunother.* **1**, 143–144.
Howell, S. B., Dean, J. H. and Law, L. W. (1975). *Int. J. Cancer*, **15**, 152–169.
Isbister, W. H., Deodhar, S. D. and Crile, G. (1971). *Transplantation*, **12**, 322–323.
Israel, L., Edelstein, R., Depieppe, A. and Dimitrov, N. (1975). *J. Natl. Cancer Inst.* **55**, 29–33.
James, S. E. and Salsbury, A. J. (1974). *Cancer Res.* **34**, 367–370.
Jurczyk-Procyk, S., Martin, M., Dubouch, P., Gheorghiu, M., Economides, F., Khalil, A. and Rappaport, H. (1976). *Cancer Immunol. Immunother.* **1**, 55–61.
Kim, U. (1970). *Science*, **167**, 72–74.
Kim, U., Baumler, A., Carruthers, C. and Bielat, K. (1975). *Proc. Nat. Acad. Sci. U.S.* **72**, 1012–1016.
Klein, G. (1975). *In* "Immunobiology of the Tumour-Host Relationship" (R. J. Smith and M. Landy, eds), p. 206. Academic Press, New York and London.
Klein, G. and Klein, E. (1977). *Transplant. Proc.* **9**, 1095–1104.
Laucius, J. F., Bodurtha, R. J., Mastrangelo, M. J. and Cree, R. M. (1974). *J. Reticuloendothelial Soc.* **16**, 347–373.
Le François, D., Youn, J. K., Belehradek, J. and Barski, G. (1971). *J. Natl. Cancer Inst.* **46**, 981–987.
Likhite, V. V. (1974a). *Cancer Res.* **34**, 2790–2794.
Likhite, V. V. (1974b). *Int. J. Cancer*, **14**, 684–690.
Martini, N., Bains, M. S. and Beattie, E. J. (1975). *Cancer*, **35**, 734–738.
Mastrangelo, M. J., Bellet, R. E., Berkelhammer, J. and Clark, W. H. (1975). *Cancer*, **36**, 1305–1308.
Mastrangelo, M. J., Berd, D. and Bellet, R. E. (1976). *Ann. N. Y. Acad. Sci.* **277**, 94–123.
Mathé, G. (1976). *Recent Results in Cancer Research*, **55**.
Mathé, G., Amiel, J. L., Schwarzenberg, L., Schneider, M., Cattan, A., Schlumberger, J. R., Hayat, M. and De Vassal, F. (1969). *Lancet*, **1**, 697–699.
Mathé, G., Weiner, R., Pouillart, P., Schwarzenberg, L., Jasmin, C., Schneider, M., Hayat, M., Amiel, J. L., De Vassal, F. and Rossenfeld, C. (1973). *Nat. Cancer Inst. Monogr.* **39**, 165–175.
Mathé, G., De Vassal, F., Delgado, M., Pouillart, P., Belpomme, D., Joseph, R., Schwarzenberg, L., Amiel, J. L., Schneider, M., Cattan, A., Musset, M., Misset, J. L. and Jasmin, C. (1976). *Cancer Immunol. Immunother.* **1**, 77–86.

McKhann, C. F. and Gunnarsson, A. (1974). *Cancer*, **34**, 1521–1531.

McKneally, M. F., Maver, C. and Kausel, H. W. (1976). *Lancet*, **1**, 377–379.

Merrin, C., Han, T., Klein, E., Wajsman, Z. and Murphy, G. P. (1975). *Cancer Chemotherapy Reps.* **59**, 157–163.

Milas, L. and Mujagic, H. (1972). *Europ. J. clin. biol. Res.* XVII, 498–500.

Milas, L. and Mujagic, H. (1973). *Int. J. Cancer*, **11**, 186–190.

Milas, L., Hunter, N., Mason, K. and Withers, H. R. (1974a). *Cancer Res.* **34**, 61–71.

Milas, L., Hunter, N. and Withers, H. R. (1974b). *Cancer Res.* **34**, 613–620.

Milas, L., Hunter, N., Basic, I. and Withers, H. R. (1974c). *J. Natl. Cancer Inst.* **52**, 1875–1880.

Milas, L., Kogelnik, H. D., Bašić, I., Mason, K., Hunter, N. and Withers, H. R. (1975). *Int. J. Cancer*, **16**, 738–746.

Moertel, C. G., Ritts, R. E., Schutt, A. J. and Hahn, R. G. (1975). *Cancer Res.* **35**, 3075–3083.

Möller, E. (1965). *J. Natl. Cancer Inst.* **35**, 1053–1059.

Moore, M., Lawrence, N. and Witherow, P. J. (1974). *Europ. J. Cancer*, **10**, 673–682.

Moore, M., Lawrence, N. and Nisbet, N. W. (1975a). *Int. J. Cancer*, **15**, 897–911.

Moore, M., Lawrence, N. and Nisbet, N. W. (1975b). *Biomedicine*, **24**, 26–31.

Morton, D. L., Eilber, F. R., Joseph, W. L., Wood, W. C., Trahan, E. and Ketcham, A. S. (1970). *Ann. Surg.* **172**, 740–749.

Morton, D. L., Eilber, F. R., Holmes, E. C., Sparks, F. C. and Ramming, K. P. (1976). *Cancer Immunol. Immunother.* **1**, 93–98.

Muggleton, P. W., Prince, G. H. and Hilton, M. L. (1975). *Lancet*, **1**, 1353–1355.

Nathanson, L. (1972). *Cancer Chemotherapy Reps.* **56**, 659–665.

Nicolson, G. L. (1976). *BBA Reviews on Cancer*, **458**, 1–72.

Nind, A. P. P., Matthews, N., Pihl, E. A., Rolland, J. M. and Nairn, R. C. (1975). *Brit. J. Cancer*, **31**, 620–630.

Old, L. J. and Boyse, E. A. (1964). *Ann. Rev. Med.* **15**, 167–179.

Paslin, D., Dimitrov, N. V. and Heaton, C. (1974). *J. Natl. Cancer Inst.* **52**, 571–573.

Penn, I. (1974). *Cancer*, **34**, 1474–1480.

Pimm, M. V. (1976). *Lancet*, **2**, 95–96.

Pimm, M. V. and Baldwin, R. W. (1975a). *Nature, Lond.* **254**, 77–78.

Pimm, M. V. and Baldwin, R. W. (1975b). *Int. J. Cancer*, **15**, 260–269.

Pimm, M. V. and Baldwin, R. W. (1976a). *Brit. J. Cancer*, **33**, 166–171.

Pimm, M. V. and Baldwin, R. W. (1976b). *Brit. J. Cancer*, **34**, 199–202.

Pimm, M. V. and Baldwin, R. W. (1976c). *Clinical Oncology*, **2**, 300–301.

Pimm, M. V. and Baldwin, R. W. (1976d). Unpublished observation.

Pimm, M. V. and Hopper, D. G. (1975). *Brit. J. Cancer*, **32**, 241–242.

Pimm, M. V., Embleton, M. J. and Baldwin, R. W. (1976). *Brit. J. Cancer*, **33**, 154–165.

Pines, A. (1976). *Lancet*, **1**, 380–381.

Pinsky, C. M., Hirshaut, Y. and Oettgen, H. F. (1973). *Nat. Cancer Inst. Monogr.* **39**, 225–228.

Pinsky, C. M., Hirshaut, Y., Wanebo, H. J., Fortner, J. G., Miké, V., Schottenfeld, D. and Oettgen, H. F. (1976) *Ann. N.Y. Acad. Sci.* **277**, 187–194.

Pinsky, C. M., Dejager, R. L., Kaufman, J., Miké, V., Hansen, J. A., Oettgen, H. F. and Krakoff, I. H. (1977). *In* "Immunotherapy of Cancer: Present Status of Trials in Man". Raven Press, New York. In press.

Pollack, S. B. (1971). *Int. J. Cancer*, **8**, 264–271.

Powles, R. L. (1976). *Brit. J. Haematol.* **32**, 145–149.

Prehn, R. T. (1969). *J. Natl. Cancer Inst.* **43**, 1215–1220.
Prehn, R. T. (1970). *J. Natl. Cancer Inst.* **45**, 1039–1045.
Prehn, R. T. (1976). *Transplant. Rev.* **28**, 34–42.
Prehn, R. T. and Lappé, M. A. (1971). *Transplant. Rev.* **7**, 26–54.
Proctor, J. W., Rudenstam, C. M. and Alexander, P. (1973). *Nature, Lond.* **242**, 29–31.
Proctor, J. W., Rudenstam, C. M. and Alexander, P. (1974). *J. Natl. Cancer Inst.* **53**, 1671–1676.
Robins, R. A. and Baldwin, R. W. (1974). *Int. J. Cancer*, **14**, 589–597.
Rowley, D. A. (1950). *J. Immunol.* **64**, 289–296.
Schwarzenberg, L., Simmler, M. C. and Pico, J. L. (1976). *Cancer Immunol. Immunother.* **1**, 69–76.
Scott, M. T. (1974). *Seminars In Oncology*, **1**, 367–378
Seigler, H. F., Shingleton, W. W., Metzgar, R. S., Buckley, C. E., Bergoc, P. M., Miller, D. S., Fetter, B. F. and Phalip, M. B. (1972). *Surgery*, **72**, 162–174.
Smith, H. G., Bast, R. C., Zbar, B. and Rapp, H. J. (1975). *J. Natl. Cancer Inst.* **55**, 1345–1352.
Spärck, J. V. (1969). *Acta Path. Microbiol. Scand.* **77**, 1–23.
Sparks, F. C., Silverstein, M. J., Hunt, J. S., Haskell, C. M., Pilch, Y. H. and Morton, D. L. (1973). *New Engl. J. Med.* **289**, 827–830.
Sparks, F. C., O'Connell, T. X., Lee, Y.-T. N. and Breeding, J. H. (1974). *J. Natl. Cancer Inst.* **53**, 1825–1829.
Stutman, O. (1975). *Advan. Cancer Res.* **22**, 261–422.
Sugarbaker, E. V. and Cohen, A. M. (1972). *Surgery*, **72**, 155–161.
Sugarbaker, E. V., Cohen, A. M. and Ketcham, A. S. (1971). *Current Topics in Surgical Res.* **3**, 349–361.
Szymaniec, S. and James, K. (1976). *Brit. J. Cancer*, **33**, 36–50.
Vaage, J. (1973). *Cancer Res.* **33**, 493–503.
Vaage, J., Chen, K. and Merrick, S. (1971). *Cancer Res.* **31**, 496–500.
Van den Brenk, H. A. S., Moore, V. and Sharpington, C. (1971). *Brit. J. Cancer*, **25**, 186–207.
Van Loveren, H. and Den Otter, W. (1974). *J. Nat. Cancer Inst.* **53**, 1057–1060.
Weston, B. J., Carter, R. L., Easty, G. C., Connell, D. I. and Davies, A. J. S. (1974). *Int. J. Cancer*, **14**, 176–185.
Wexler, H., Chretien, P. B., and Ketcham, A. S. (1972). *J. Natl. Cancer Inst.* **48**, 657–663.
Wexler, H., Chretien, P. B., Ketcham, A. S. and Sindelar, W. F. (1975). *Cancer*, **36**, 2042–2047.
Woodruff, M. F. A. and Dunbar, N. (1975). *Brit. J. Cancer*, **32**, 34–41.
Yuhas, J. M. and Pazmiño, N. H. (1974). *Cancer Res.* **34**, 2005–2010.
Yuhas, J. M., Pazmiño, N. H., Proctor, J. O. and Toya, R. E. (1974). *Cancer Res.* **34**, 722–728.
Zarling, J. M. and Tevethia, S. S. (1973). *J. Natl. Cancer Inst.* **50**, 137–147.
Zbar, B. and Tanaka, T. (1971). *Science*, **172**, 271–273.
Zbar, B., Bernstein, I. D., Bartlett, G. L., Hanna, M. G., Jr. and Rapp, H. J. (1972). *J. Natl. Cancer Inst.* **49**, 119–130.

Chapter *VII*

The Chemotherapy of Metastatic Disease

STEPHEN K. CARTER

Northern California Cancer Research Program, Palo Alto, California 94304 U.S.A.

I. Introduction

The chemotherapy of metastatic disease can be looked at in a variety of ways. There is the chemotherapy which is directed at clinically evident metastatic disease which is the traditional role for drugs in the therapy of solid tumors; there is also chemotherapy which is directed at microscopic metastatic disease which is the presumed cause of failure after curative intent therapy with surgery and radiotherapy. It is the purpose of this paper to review the principles of clinical cancer chemotherapy against both kinds of metastatic disease and to give a broad overview of the current status of these approaches against the major solid tumors.

The basic assumption in cancer treatment is that all malignant cells should be destroyed, removed, or neutralized to achieve cure. In practice, five therapy modalities have this potential and, therefore, are widely used. They are: surgery, radiotherapy, chemotherapy, endocrinotherapy, and possibly immunotherapy. Some modalities are more successful than others, but all are incompletely understood and all are subject to improvements in their research concept and widespread application.

Chemotherapy is a relatively infant science compared to surgery and radiation, but has already been successful in reducing the mortality in a number of different diseases. Drugs alone can cure significant numbers of patients with some forms of cancer, such as choriocarcinoma and Burkitt's lymphoma. There are other cancers (e.g. acute lymphocytic leukemia, Hodgkin's disease, histiocytic lymphomas, Ewing's tumor, Wilms' tumor, embryonal rhabdomyosarcoma, testicular tumors, and retinoblastoma) in which chemotherapy, either alone or in combination with other modalities, can bring about normal life expectancy in a significant percentage of patients with advanced disease. The percentage of patients achieving normal life expectancy ranges from about 90% in Wilms' tumor to about 15% in metastatic testicular tumor.

Cancer can be classified into two major categories: solid tumors and hematologic malignancies. Solid tumors are initially confined to specific tissue or organ sites. In time, however, cancer cells break off from the original tumor mass, enter the blood or lymph system, reach distant parts of the body, and start secondary growths there (metastasis); when this occurs, the disease is in the disseminated stage. Conversely, hematologic malignancies involve the blood and lymph systems, and for this reason, they are frequently disseminated diseases from the very beginning.

In solid tumors, surgery and/or radiotherapy are the traditional, primarily chosen treatments. Neither modality, however, can be considered curative once disease has metastasised beyond the local region (primary site and nearby lymph nodes) or has involved a vital organ extensively. Chemotherapy is relegated almost exclusively to secondary or tertiary treatment of solid tumors, i.e. when surgery and radiotherapy fail. Conversely, in hematologic malignancies, chemotherapy is the treatment of choice at diagnosis.

Since the highest curative potential for solid tumors exists when the tumor is both small and localized, early detection offers the best opportunity for control. However, at the time of initial diagnosis, a number of patients already have extensive disease which local treatment modalities (surgery and/or radiotherapy) cannot cure. Alternatively, by the time of primary therapy, some other patients have established microscopic foci of metastatic disease which available diagnostic techniques cannot detect and local treatment modalities cannot remove or destroy. In this case, it erroneously appears that the tumor is still localized. Relapses after surgery and/or radiotherapy are largely attributable to metastatic spread initiated prior to treatment. This is not to deny, however, that in certain situations reinduction of additional primary tumor growths at other anatomical sites could be responsible for the reappearance of the disease.

II. Basic Concepts in Cancer Chemotherapy

All living things have an inherent capacity to multiply and they cease multiplication for a variety of reasons. In complex cellular organizations (such as man) a cellular "brake" is required to prevent overgrowth for the benefit of the community of cells. This appears to be controlled by an unknown feedback mechanism probably resulting from contact phenomena when cells are crowded. In cancerous growth, cells no longer cease multiplying when they reach a critical mass and the uncontrolled growth leads to the death of the host. In the early phases of growth, tumor cells grow exponentially but as tumor mass increases the time it takes a tumor to double its volume increases: this is best described as a gompertzian function. It is likely

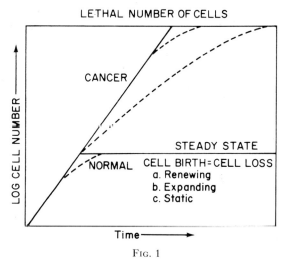

FIG. 1

that such changes in tumor doubling time are somehow related to crowding and loss of nutrient supply via the vascular system. Three broad mechanisms have been postulated to explain the prolonged volume doubling time: (a) an increase in cell cycle time (the time from one mitosis to the next); (b) a decrease in the growth fraction (cells participating in cell division in the mass); and (c) an increase in cell loss from the tumor as it ages.

The utilization of drugs in the treatment of cancer is to achieve the selective killing of tumor cells. This is based on the cell-kill hypothesis as elucidated by Skipper and his colleagues (1964). The principles of the hypothesis (as worked out in L1210 leukemia) are as follows: (a) the survival of an animal with leukemia is inversely related to either the number of leukemic cells inoculated or the number remaining after treatment; (b) a single leukemia cell is capable of multiplying and eventually killing the host; (c) for most drugs, a clear relationship exists between the drug dose and its ability to eradicate tumor cells within the limits of toxicity to the host; (d) a given dose of a drug kills a constant fraction of cells, not a constant number, regardless of the cell numbers present at the time of therapy. This means that cell destruction by drugs follows first-order kinetics. A treatment reducing a population from 1,000,000 to 10 cells should reduce a population of 100,000 to 1 cell. The implications of the fractional cell killing effect is that, to eradicate a tumor population effectively, it is necessary either to increase the dose of drug or drugs within limits tolerated by the host, or to start treatment when the number of cells is small enough to allow tumor destruction at reasonably tolerated doses. The implication is not, as has been often stated, that eradication of the last neoplastic cell is not possible with chemotherapy.

Contrary to popular opinion among physicians, the cytotoxicity of cancer chemotherapeutic agents has a definite selectivity for cancer cells over the normal host cells. This is well illustrated by using a dual spleen colony assay to quantitate the survival of lymphoma and normal cells in animal systems. Work in these systems has shown that, for some agents, as much as 10,000-times greater cell kill of lymphoma over marrow cells is achieved (Holland and Glidewell, 1970). The major reason for the selectivity of this system is most likely due to proliferative differences.

The effectiveness of an anti-tumor agent is dependent on a mixture of factors which can be divided broadly into kinetic factors and pharmacologic factors.

It is now well-established that all renewing cells that are synthesizing DNA go through a series of phases. At the completion of mitosis (M), the cells spend a variable period of time in a resting phase (G_1). During G, DNA synthesis for cell replication apparently is absent but does proceed for repair purposes, and RNA and protein synthesis continue normally. (3) In late G (the G–S conversion), an unknown signal initiates a burst of RNA synthesis and shortly thereafter the DNA synthetic period (S phase) begins and the cell is committed to either undergo division or remain polypoid. Next, the cells cease DNA synthesis during the G_2 phase before entry into mytosis, although RNA and protein synthesis continue; then in mitosis the rates of protein and RNA synthesis diminish abruptly while the genetic material is segregated into daughter cells. An additional resting phase (G_0) of the cell cycle has also been described: these are the cells which, although not in cycle, are capable of proliferation and they constitute the cells which are for the most part refractory to cancer chemotherapeutic agents.

Tumor growth is dependent on the proliferating pool (growth fraction) of cells in the tumor mass. This concept of the proliferation pool or growth fraction was introduced by Mendelsohn (Peters, 1971). This work was intensively followed up by Skipper and his colleagues (1964). Their work can briefly be summarized as follows: the rate of growth of doubling time of small tumors is largely, but not entirely, dependent upon the percentage of cells in the mitotic cycle. Particularly in larger tumors, rate of growth is also contingent on the number of tumor cells spontaneously dying, or perhaps, becoming differentiated.

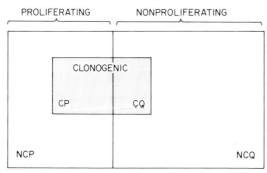

- CP   are clonogenic proliferating cells
- CQ   are clonogenic nonproliferating cells (G_0 cells)
- NCP are nonclonogenic proliferating cells (doomed cells)
- NCQ are nonclonogenic nonproliferating cells (end cells)

Fig. 2

The cell types in any individual tumor mass can be, based on the above, represented in four compartments (Fig. 2). Most likely, tumor cell populations resemble a renewing population of normal cells. Some cell differentiation may be associated with inability to divide beyond one or two cell divisions and tumor cells would be continually renewed from the tumor stem cell or clonogenic pool. Such a model would explain current cytokinetic information and would suggest that cancer cells are not totally unresponsive to growth control mechanisms.

Cell-population kinetics provide one approach to understanding drug susceptibility in some tumors. Tumors may be proliferating more rapidly than normal cell populations or tumor cells may have more cells in the drug sensitive phases of the cell cycle. This does not, however, explain all successes and failures of drug therapy.

Another reason for success or failure is related to pharmacologic disposition of drugs in patients. Even if the tumor is susceptible to a drug, it cannot influence the tumor in a favorable way unless the drug reaches the tumor site and remains there in tumoricidal concentration for a long enough period to kill the tumor cells. In general, the purpose of pharmacology studies is to tell the physician how to get effective concentrations (C) of drug to the target site for a long enough time (T) to bring about the desired effect. This is often referrred to as the optimal C × T, and, in most diseases, this can be approximated for man by studies in animals of the delivery of drug to the organs and tissues of interest. What makes cancer different is the need to relate optimal

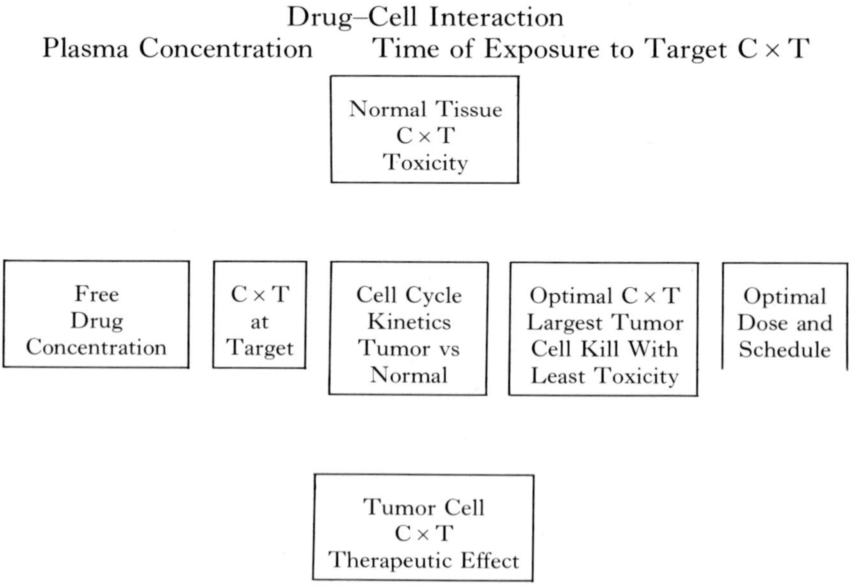

Drug–Cell Interaction
Plasma Concentration   Time of Exposure to Target C × T

Normal Tissue C × T Toxicity

Free Drug Concentration	C × T at Target	Cell Cycle Kinetics Tumor vs Normal	Optimal C × T Largest Tumor Cell Kill With Least Toxicity	Optimal Dose and Schedule

Tumor Cell C × T Therapeutic Effect

FIG. 3. An ideal scheme of the relationship between the cellular kinetics of normal and tumor tissue and the effective blood levels of antitumor agents

$C \times T$ to the phases of the cell cycle. First, the optimal $C \times T$ for the tumor must be estimated for the real target—the tumor cells that are susceptible to killing by the drug. Secondly, the calculation of optimal $C \times T$ for the safety of the patient (e.g. the $C \times T$ that will be tolerable for the bone marrow or gastrointestinal cells in most cases) must reckon with the percentage of normal cells that are at risk by being in DNA synthesis, mitosis or any other susceptible phase. Another important factor to consider is that the cell population kinetics of both tumor cells and normal cells are perturbed as a result of drug administration so that after the perturbation the size of the growth fraction and, therefore, the potential for drug effect is altered. Understanding the failures of active drugs to cause regression of cancer will depend to a significant extent upon successful delineation of this complex pharmacology.

This is all summarized in Fig. 3. The effectiveness of an anti-tumor agent is directly related to its $C \times T$ which is markedly affected by dose and schedule. The tumor cell, and to some degree the critical normal tissues, present variable and fluctuating targets. Knowledge of cell kinetics of normal tissue, which should remain relatively constant, and of tumor populations, can help determine the most effective means of obtaining an optimum $C \times T$ by the most appropriate doses and schedules. The optimum $C \times T$ should kill the maximum tumor cells with minimal lethality in cells of normal tissue.

The potential circumvention of resistance to treatment has, historically, probably been the most important factor prompting studies of drug combinations. Human tumors, in contrast to many

Mechanism	Example
1. Insufficient drug uptake by cancer cell	Methotrexate Daunomycin
2. Insufficient activation of drug	6-Mercaptopurine 5-Fluorouracil
3. Increased inactivation	Cytosine Arabinoside
4. Increased concentration of a target enzyme	Methotrexate
5. Decreased requirement for a specific metabolic product	L-Asparaginase
6. Increased utilization of an alternate biochemical pathway (Salvage)	Anti-metabolites
7. Rapid repair of a drug induced lesion	Alkylating Agents

Fig. 4. Resistance to anticancer drugs

animal tumors, present with a greatly reduced percentage of cells in the proliferating pool. Effective chemotherapy is in most cases required to be repeated therapy over long intervals. Under these circumstances, repetitive exposure of tumor cells to chemicals can lead to clinical resistance to drugs. The clinician is faced with a two-fold problem: the re-growth of tumor cells between cycles of therapy (which must be separated by intervals sufficient to allow recovery of normal tissues): and reduced amounts of tumor-cell kill with subsequent cycles of treatment owing to the development of resistant cell lines. Largely on the basis of experimental systems, various mechanisms have been proposed for the development of resistance and are summarized in Fig. 4. Drug resistance can be the result of step-wise induction or related to the presence of a population of organisms inherently resistant to the drug employed. If such a mechanism for resistance exists in cancer-cell populations (as it does for bacterial populations), additional effective drugs may be required for each distinct resistant cell line until the number of viable cells can be reduced to zero or an effective zero (a small enough number of cells to be controlled by the host's own defence mechanisms). The success of any drug treatment will be dependent on the number of resistant lines in the tumor population and the number of available drugs that can be used effectively in combination. In addition to cellular mechanisms of resistance, host factors might lead to diminished sensitivity of the tumor. An example would be reduced concentration of active drug reaching the tumor cells.

Two conceptual approaches to the design of clinical combinations have been described. One approach is biochemical (DeVita *et al.*, 1970). Combinations of drugs can be designed with agents that produce different biochemical lesions so as to attack multiple sites in

TESTING NEW DRUGS AND DRUG COMBINATIONS IN ADVANCED
DISEASE

DEVELOPING OPTIMUM CHEMOTHERAPY FOR PRIMARY
TREATMENT OF DISSEMINATED DISEASE

INTEGRATING OPTIMUM CHEMOTHERAPY INTO A COMBINED
MODALITY APPROACH FOR PRIMARY TREATMENT OF LOCAL AND
REGIONAL DISEASE

FIG. 5

biosynthetic pathways or inhibit several processes involved in maintenance and function of essential macromolecules. The common goal is to decrease the production and availability of a specific end-product vital for tumor-cell growth and replication. Three basic schemes have been described; the inhibition of different enzymatic steps in a biochemical pathway leading to the production of an essential metabolite has been designated sequential blockage. The simultaneous inhibition of parallel metabolic pathways involved in the synthesis of a common end-product has been termed concurrent blockage. Complementary inhibition envisions the selection of agents that produce biochemical lesions at different loci in the synthesis of polymeric molecules.

Although this type of approach to the design of drug combinations is intellectually satisfying, it is recognized that such biochemical considerations are not always predictive of biological synergism and, in particular, that they do not estimate the degree of depletion of the specific end-product required for tumor cell destruction; it also assumes selective toxicity for the tumor tissue. None of the successful combinations in usage today have been developed purely as the result of this approach; nevertheless, it is quite possible that some of them owe their effectiveness, in part, to such synergistic mechanisms.

The *sine qua non* of successful combined drug programs has been the use of drugs that are individually active in the specific disease when used alone. In line with this the tumors successfully treated with combinations have generally been the ones designated as "drug sensitive": this means that several effective drugs were available that acted by different mechanisms. When several choices of drugs were available within a class of agents, drug selection was guided by the type of dose-limiting toxicity likely to be produced by other agents employed in the combination. Selections made in this fashion have allowed anti-tumor agents to be used in combination in nearly full clinical dosage, an apparent requirement, at least for some combinations.

Another facet of successful combination has been the application of intermittent treatment schedules which enable a greater intensity of treatment to be applied. One theoretical advantage to this is that if the combination exerts a selective killing effect on tumor over normal bone marrow, an interval of two to three weeks between courses is usually sufficient to allow recovery of the marrow to pretreatment levels. An additional bonus of intermittent scheduling is the potential recovery of the host's immunologic mechanism between exposures to cycles of chemotherapy (Holland and Hreshchyshyn, 1967).

III. Combined Modality Treatment

Curative surgical and radiological intervention is possible in man, only if metastatic spread from the primary tumor has not yet occurred. Since 50% or more of malignant tumors of man may have metastasised prior to clinical recognition, they may be beyond the reach of curative surgical or radiologic treatment when they initially present. Metastatic tumor cell foci of $\leq 10^9$ cells, particularly if widely disseminated are, in the main, grossly undetectable and are, therefore, a target for chemotherapy (Holland and Hreshchyshyn, 1967).

Estimations have been made of the likely total body burden of viable tumor remaining after surgery and/or radiation therapy has removed all clinically visible or detectable tumor foci (Holland et al., 1971). These estimates are based on the indicated probability that each gram of tumor may contain as many as 10^9 cells (Brewer et al., 1970; Mackenzie, 1966). A single metastatic focus, 1 mm in diameter, may contain 10^5–10^6 tumor cells and this number will range downward to one cell with progressively smaller metastases. The number and size of these micrometastases will determine the likely requirements for cure. It is highly variable, but in many cases the total tumor cell population in unrecognized metastases may be very large and formidable, especially if reduction to small number (perhaps zero) may be required for cure.

The conceptual design of chemotherapy utilization in this situation is based on first-order kinetics of drug kill and the understanding of tumor cell population kinetics described earlier. It has been repeatedly shown that the time duration of the division cycle (T_c) of tumor cells, in a wide range of systems, is directly related to tumor mass—the larger the tumor cell population, the longer the division cycle time (T_c) (Carter, 1975; Sullivan and Sutow, 1969; Sutow et al., 1970; Farber, 1964; Skipper et al., 1964).

Reduction of total body burden of tumor cells by an effective but non-curative therapy has been shown to shorten the T_c in both acute lymphoblastic leukemia (Pratt et al., 1972) and ovarian cancer (Wilbur et al., 1971). In experimental systems, it has been shown that the T_c of micrometastases is significantly shorter than that of cells in the primary tumor (in the same host) which shed the tumor cells to the metastases (Ellsworth, 1968). Reduction in total body burden of tumor cells has been shown to decrease the tumor mass doubling time with sarcoma 180 and adenocarcinoma 755 in mice (Hustu et al., 1968). All of this leads to the implication that drugs will achieve increased cell kill to tumor cell populations as tumor burden is reduced.

The principles of tumor population kinetics and the first-order kinetics of drug kill indicate that (a) chemotherapy as an adjuvant to either surgical or radiological therapy should be started as soon as possible after the primary treatment, and (b) that drugs which have the ability to kill tumor cells in the advanced (clinically visible) state should be even more effective when utilized to treat micrometastatic disease.

In line with the above a broad overall strategy for increasing cure rates in solid tumors which involves integration of chemotherapy into combined modalities for primary treatment has been developed (Carter and Soper, 1974). The single drugs or drug combinations showing positive results in advanced disease will be moved into primary treatment of disseminated disease; then, the optimal drug regimens evolved in this situation will be integrated with other modalities into combined modality therapy for primary treatment of local and regional disease.

The current status of chemotherapy in some of the common solid tumors will be outlined in the following sections.

A. *Breast Cancer*

The treatment of advanced breast cancer is a sequential mixture of hormonal and cytotoxic therapy which varies from patient to patient depending upon the variables of: (1) menstrual status; (2) age; (3) disease-free interval after surgical treatment; (4) extent and location of metastases; (5) rapidity of tumor growth, and (6) previous response of metastatic disease to hormonal manipulation. No standard regimen exists for treating every patient with disseminated breast cancer, but most clinicians divide women into three broad categories based on menopausal status and proceed on to treatment sequences which utilize initial hormonal therapy of some type unless the disease involves lymphangitic pulmonary metastases, symptomatic liver metastases or some evidence of rapid growth. These categories are:

(1) Menstruating women.
(2) Those who have not had a menstrual period for the last six months to five years.
(3) Women who are more than five years post-menopausal.

Castration is the usual therapy for the pre-menopausal women. In most treatment centers surgical oophorectomy is preferred over radiation castration: this approach yields responses of 20 to 40%; the best responses occur in women from 35 to 45 years of age. Younger women, and those with rapidly progressive disease, should be treated initially with chemotherapy, since they are less likely to benefit from this procedure. The pre-menopausal women who respond to castration have a reasonable likelihood of responding to a second hormonal treatment. Some clinicians prefer the additive use of androgens while others lean toward the surgical ablative procedures of either bilateral adrenalectomy or hypophysectomy. A cogent argument can also be made to utilize chemotherapy at this time, since the response rates in the literature are higher than those reported for secondary hormonal treatment. The pre-menopausal woman who fails to respond to oophorectomy has a poor prognosis and chemotherapy should be the next therapy attempted.

Women six months to five years post-menopausal are a difficult group in which to prescribe treatment. Castration gives a low response rate as does additive hormonal treatment. The utilization of chemotherapy for initial treatment is one valid alternative in this situation. The major ablative procedures can be done initially with castration added to adrenalectomy and the reported response rate is about 30%. Chemotherapy gives comparable to higher response rates although with a somewhat shorter duration of remission. Patients with liver metastases do poorly with ablative procedures and should go initially to chemotherapy. The best group in which to consider this approach is the women who have relatively slow-going bone metastases or advanced local disease with a free-interval of more than two years duration.

The traditional approach to women more than five years post-menopausal is therapy with estrogens. The older the patient the higher the potential response, and in women over 70 with predominant cutaneous or lymph node metastases the response rate may approach 50%. Androgens can also be used and for women with bone metastases may be equal to estrogens. In this group of patients also, chemotherapy response rates are higher and a valid approach could be to utilize chemotherapy from the initial point of relapse.

Breast cancer is responsible to a wide range of single agents. The most commonly used single agents are the alkylating agents (cyclophosphamide, L-phenylalanine mustard, thio-tepa, chlorambucil), 5-Fluorouracil and Adriamycin. Adriamycin, which is the newest agent to be uncovered with activity in breast cancer, has the highest reported response rates among the single agents which are in excess of 40% in patients not previously treated with chemotherapy. Other agents with activity but rarely used a primary treatment, include the vinca alkaloids and methotrexate. Prednisone and other adrenocortical steroids often produce subjective and occasionally ($\sim 20\%$) objective responses of a short duration. In general, complete responses with single agents are uncommon and the average duration of response is in the range of three to four months which is shorter than that observed with hormonal treatment.

As discussed earlier, some of the prerequisites for drugs to be used in a successful combination approach to a given tumor are: (a) the drugs should be active as single agents; (b) the drugs should have independent mechanisms of action, and (c) the drugs should not produce overlapping toxicity: most of these conditions can be met in the chemotherapy of breast cancer. A number of drugs with differing mechanisms of action, such as cyclophosphamide, methotrexate, 5-fluorouracil, and vincristine, have significant activity as single agents. Although there is some degree of overlapping toxicity, the potential clearly exists for combination regimens employing doses of significant therapeutic potential.

In 1969, Cooper presented the results of a 5-drug combination utilizing: Cyclophosphamide, Methotrexate, 5-Fluorouracil, Vincristine, Prednisone. He reported a 90% complete remission rate in a group of 60 hormone-resistant patients with far-advanced breast cancer (Carter, S. K., 1972, 1974; Broder and Tormey, 1974).

A wide range of combinations have evolved from the Cooper 5-drug regimen and which have utilized Adriamycin and have been tested over the last several years. It is clear from all of these studies that in experienced hands combination chemotherapy can give response rates of about 50% with average durations of remission in the 7- to 9-month range. This is significantly less than reported by Cooper but significantly higher than reported for single agents or hormones. No single combination can be definitely recommended but four of the most commonly and easily used regimens are listed in Fig. 6. Active investigation is on-going to improve the therapeutic indices of combinations and to test whether the addition of hormonal treatment or immunotherapy to the combinations will be a valuable endeavour. The results of these studies are not yet available and, therefore, at this point in time these approaches cannot be recommended for general use.

It is clear that combination chemotherapy can produce impressive response rates, although in every case these appear to be less than the additive effect of each component drug used optimally alone. Much work still remains to be done in elucidating the optimum drug combinations and sequences of drug administration. At this point no individual combination can be recommended as optimal and the

I. CMF

Cyclophosphamide	$100 \ mg/m^2/d \times 14$	Repeat
Methotrexate	$40 \ mg/m^2/d$ 1 & 8	every
5-Fluorouracil	$600 \ mg/m^2/d$ 1–8	28 days

II. CFP

Cyclophosphamide	$4 \ mg/kg/d \times 5$	Repeat
5-Fluorouracil	$8 \ mg/kg/d \times 5$	every
Prednisone	$30 \ mg/d \times 14$ then taper	28 days

III. CMFVP ("Cooper" Regimen)

Cyclophosphamide	$2 \ mg/kg/d$
Methotrexate	$0.75 \ mg/kg/wk$
5-Fluorouracil	$12 \ mg/kg/wk$
Vincristine	$0.25 \ mcg/kg/wk$
Prednisone	$0.75 \ mg/kg/d \times 21$ then taper

IV. AC

| Adriamycin | $40 \ mg/m^2$ | Repeat every |
| Cyclophosphamide | $500 \ mg/m^2$ | 28 days |

Fig. 6. Effective combination regimens for disseminated breast cancer

definitive value of combinations over sequential use of single agents for palliating advanced disease remains to be established. Despite this, the cell-kill potential of combinations as evidenced by remission induction figures appears to be higher and makes this approach highly attractive for use in combined modality regimens.

Breast cancer is one area where the combined modality approach is yielding some positive results in preliminary investigations. In early studies, Nissen-Mayer et al., of the Scandinavian Adjuvant Chemotherapy Study Group and Fisher et al. (1975) in the United States reported improved survival among patients having operable breast cancer treated by short courses of chemotherapy. Both studies were based on the concept that tumor cells are disseminated at the time of surgery and metastases can be prevented by early chemotherapy. The Scandinavian group observed improved survival at six years after using only a short course of post-operative cyclophosphamide. Fisher and his associates noted a significant decrease in recurrence rates after a single course of thiotepa in pre-menopausal women having four or more positive lymph nodes. More recently, this group reported that a 20% improvement in survival notes at five years has persisted for ten years (Carter, S. K., 1974).

The rationale of employing chemotherapy as a surgical adjuvant has evolved significantly during the past 15 years. The earlier practice of limiting chemotherapy to use during surgery or in an immediate post-operative course (in hopes of killing the circulating tumor cell) has been replaced by more extensive courses of drug treatment. Two recent studies illustrate how a longer period of adjuvant chemotherapy has significantly delayed disease recurrence in breast cancer.

Fisher *et al.* (1975) have reported their findings in a study conducted at 37 hospitals using L-PAM (Melphalan) at dose of 0·15 mg/kg/day for five days post-operatively in patients having positive nodes after mastectomy: the study included 250 patients. The data at two years indicated that the recurrence rate was significantly reduced in patients who received the chemotherapy. Results were particularly striking in pre-menopausal women where tumor recurrence occurred in only 1 of 30 who received the drug, compared to 11 of 37 who only had surgery. Recurrence rates also were reduced among post-menopausal women treated with L-PAM but not as markedly as in the pre-menopausal group.

The second study was conducted by Bonadonna and his associates at the Instituto Nazional Tumori in Milan, Italy (Carter, S. K., 1974). Using the same stratification of patients and eligibility criteria employed by Fisher *et al.*, they allocated patients with positive nodes after mastectomy to receive a 3-drug combination of "CMF" (cyclo-phosphamide, methotrexate, and 5-fluorouracil) or the surgery alone. In 18 months of patient accural, 114 patients have been entered on surgery alone and 87 are in the "CMF" study arm. Fourteen patients (12%) have relapsed on surgery alone versus 1 patient (1%) treated by "CMF" and surgery.

More recent follow-up analysis of these studies has shown that in post-menopausal women the data are no longer significantly positive. It is clear that the claims made for the early analysis will have to be interpreted with caution until longer follow-up is available (Jaffe *et al.*, 1974; Cortes, *et al.*, 1974; Sutow *et al.*, 1975).

B. *Large Bowel*

5-Fluorouracil (5-FU) is the standard single agent for the therapy of advanced large bowel cancer. An overall response rate of 20% has been observed. The most commonly utilized approach to administering 5-FU is the loading course schedule in which the drug is given daily for five days and then possibly every other day for several additional doses. A wide range of additional approaches have been devised for administering the drug, including 2-, 8-, and 24-hour infusions, administration by weekly injection or by intensive course followed by weekly injection administration in 5% or 10% dextrose, and oral use in capsules or liquid form. There is considerable evidence that a change in the duration of frequency of administration alters the intensity of the overall pharmacologic effect of 5-FU, but no definitive evidence that this is accompanied by a therapeutic index superior to that of the loading course approach.

One of the latest approaches to 5-FU therapy has involved a resurgence of interest in oral administration. The Mayo Clinic group recently performed a double blind study comparing the oral and intravenous route. With the oral route, twice the dose was required to reach a degree of marrow toxicity equal to that induced by rapid injection. The oral drug also produced a higher incidence of gastro-intestinal toxicity. After 10 weeks the response rate was only 9% for the oral route compared to 21% for the parenteral approach. The duration of response was also significantly shorter with the oral drug. These results did not change when patients with metastatic disease in the liver were analyzed separately. When the clinical pharmacology was compared, the blood levels of 5-FU given orally were substantially more erratic than they were after i.v. administration. At this point the oral approach cannot be recommended for routine usage.

The only other standard available drug with evidence of activity in colorectal cancer, is Mitomycin C which was originally isolated and developed in Japan. A review of the Japanese literature has shown 50 regressions in 154 patients with gastro-intestinal cancer. At the Mayo Clinic in the U.S. only six objective regressions in 56 patients with large bowel cancer were observed and these were of short duration. Although the drug is capable of inducing regressions in large bowel cancer, its marked potential for marrow toxicity and the hazard of infiltration ulcers limits its use.

Among investigational agents, the nitrosources developed in the USA have shown some level of activity. Studies in the Mayo Clinic have shown response rates of 12·5% (8/64) with BCNU, 10% (7/75) with CCNU and 17·5% (7/40) with methyl-CCNU. The Mayo Clinic, with methyl-CNU in a randomized comparison with 5-FU, has shown the new drug to be at least equal to, or perhaps slightly better, than the standard fluorinated pyrimidine. Another compound, Razoxane ICRF-159 has also shown a response rate of 12% in U.S. studies.

In the past few years various drug combinations were tested in the search for more effective chemotherapy of gastro-intestinal cancer. One combination MIFUCA (Mitomycin C, Cytosine Arabinoside, and 5-FU), was investigated initially in Japan with some reports of increased activity. However, results in colon carcinoma at Memorial Sloan Kettering Hospital, New York, showed no significant improvement over those achieved with 5-FU alone. Results with work at the Mayo Clinic on large bowel cancer have indicated that combinations of 5-FU + BCNU, 5-FU + Mitomycin C, or Mitomycin C + BCNU do not offer any advantage in therapeutic response over 5-FU used alone. A recently completed study, however, indicated that the combination 5-FU + MeCCNU + Vincristine may produce objective responses in advanced colorectal cancer significantly superior to those obtained with 5-FU. In a controlled study, a 43·5% objective response rate was obtained with this combination compared to only 19% with 5-FU alone, but survival was not significantly different in both groups. Studies are on-going to determine whether such combinations can be routinely recommended.

Studies utilizing 5-FU as an adjuvant to surgery in the hope of eradicating the microscopic foci of metastatic disease remaining after surgery, have not been significantly successful and this approach cannot be routinely recommended. Currently, vigorous investigation therapeutic setting (Carter, S. K., 1976; Moertel et al., 1975; Baker et al., 1975; Moertel, 1975).

C. Gastric Cancer

The two major drugs which are commonly utilized to treat gastric cancer are 5-Fluorouracil and Mitomycin C. 5-Fluorouracil is the most extensively studied single agent for the treatment of gastric carcinoma. The most common dose schedule has been the loading course, in which the drug was originally administered i.v. at 15 mg/kg/day × 5, followed by half-doses every other day until toxicity occurred. The maintenance schedules vary from weekly to bi-weekly doses to monthly loading courses. Recently, a large randomized study in carcinoma of the colon and breast has shown that response rates and duration are equivalent for a single weekly vs. monthly loading course maintenance regimens. The weekly maintenance schedule is said to offer the benefit of better tolerance and acceptability.

Controversy still exists concerning the optimum method for administering 5-FU. The standard loading-course method was attended by a high risk of severe toxicity and acute drug-related deaths. Several variations of the loading course have evolved. Currently, the Mayo Clinic group is employing a 5-day course of 13·5 mg/kg repeated every 5 weeks, with therapy interrupted if stomatitis or diarrhea develops. Using this regimen the drug-related mortality rate is reportedly less than 1%.

Studies have shown that 5-FU added to radiotherapy can enhance survival in patients with locally unresectable disease. The overall objective with 5-FU is 20–25% with an average four to five months duration of response. In spite of the relatively large number of patients treated with 5-FU, there has rarely been a systematic analysis of factors such as age, sex, disease-free interval, histologic grade of the tumor, or sites of metastasis, which might predispose to a favorable or unfavorable response.

In Japan the most commonly utilized drug is Mitomycin C and it has been the second most frequently used drug in the United States. The daily schedule of administration has proven to have marked toxicity, a narrow therapeutic index and a potential for delayed and persistent hetatopoetic toxicity. The utilization of either a low protracted dose schedule or large intermittent doses has led to more manageable levels of toxicity.

Mitomycin C generally causes delayed cumulative toxicity, which probably explains the difficulty in giving prolonged courses and favors use of a high intermittent schedule where the toxicity observed in one course can be used to adjust the dose in subsequent courses. Renal toxicity has been described and may be more pronounced with the high intermittent dose schedule.

The over all objective response rate is between 20–30% with the higher response rates being reported in Japanese data. The average duration of response ranges from 1–3 months.

The nitrosoureas (BCNU, CCNU and methyl-CCNU) have shown some evidence of activity. BCNU has yielded an objective response rate of 18% (6/33) and an average duration of response of 4·5 months in gastric cancer patients, most of whom had no prior therapy. Recently evidence of activity has been seen with Adriamycin with an approximate response rate of 25%.

Combination approaches have been more successful in stomach cancer than in any other gastro-intestinal neoplasm. The Japanese have reported higher response rates with a combination of 5-FU, Mitomycin C and Cytosine Arabinoside. The therapeutic activity of this combination has been confirmed at the Memorial Sloan-Kettering Cancer Center. The Mayo Clinic has observed a 41% response rate with the combination of 5-FU + BCNU with survival superior to a concomitant control of both single agents. More recently the combination of 5-FU and methyl CCNU is also showing these high response rates.

The utilization of chemotherapy as an adjuvant to surgery has been extensively evaluated in Japan, the USSR and the USA. The Japanese have studied predominately Mitomycin C alone or in combination. While a few results are positive, most studies have not show a meaningful survival gain.

In the United States, studies with thiotepa and FUDR have all been negative but all utilized short-term regimens of chemotherapy. Current trials involve long-term administration of methyl CCNU plus 5-FU.

The past experience with surgical adjuvant chemotherapy neither confirms nor denies the utility of this approach. However, this lack of a definitive answer, which is largely due to faulty study designs, and possibly to inadequate chemotherapy, does permit some insight into certain principles that may be critical in designing future combined modality therapies published to date (Moertel, 1975; Comis and Carter, S. K., 1974a, 1974b).

D. Lung Cancer

Bronchogenic carcinoma is now the most common malignancy among men in many countries and the leading cause of death from cancer in that group. The data in over 22,000 cases analysed from 1955 to 1964 show that only 21% of the patients could receive a surgical resection at the time of diagnosis. In this group the overall 5-year survival rate was 7% with an observed median survival time (MST) of 0·4 years. For 4193 cases that were localized at diagnosis, the 5-year survival was 24% with a 1·1 year MST. Unfortunately, the percentage of cases with localized disease at diagnosis has remained stable since 1940.

The situation is truly dismal in patients who are considered inoperable at the time of diagnosis. The Veterans Administration Lung Cancer Study Group of the U.S. has reported an analysis by extent of disease as well as histologic type, in a series of inoperable patients who received only supportive therapy. Patients with tumor clinically confined to one hemithorax (i.e. within the confines of a single radiotherapy portal) were termed as having "limited" disease and all others as "extensive" disease. In 130 patients with limited disease, the MST was 15·7 weeks from the time the patient was deemed inoperable, while in extensive disease the MST was 9·4 weeks.

Efforts to improve these dismal results by radiotherapy and chemotherapy have so far met with very limited success. Patients with limited disease may experience some improvement in survival from radiotherapy alone. A large-scale randomized study of radiation therapy versus placebo, showed that treated patients survived about

20% longer than untreated controls. The effect of radiotherapy on limited disease may be particularly true for the squamous cell types, with MST of 60 weeks in such patients, versus 25 weeks in a group receiving single-drug therapy in one recent study. However, other studies have failed to demonstrate improved survival, even in limited disease, for patients receiving radiotherapy.

Oat cell (USC) carcinoma accounts for 15–20% of diagnosed cases of lung cancer. Because of the prevalence of lung cancer, it is therefore a relatively common disease. Most thoracic surgeons today feel that patients with this histological diagnosis should not undergo an attempt at curative resection, since even those with clinically limited disease usually have microscopic dissemination. Radiation therapy alone has been reported to produce long-term (more than 5 years) disease-free survival in 4% of patients with clinically limited disease, but *median* survival in such patients treated with radiotherapy was no better than survival on no specific treatment, in a randomized trial (3 months). This lack of effect on survival was found in spite of the fact that the tumor is radiation-sensitive: objective regression of tumor mass by $> 50\%$ occurs in the majority with response rates as high as 82% reported (Carter and Livingston, 1973). The early dissemination, radiation sensitivity, and short survial characteristic of USC carcinoma are all probably related to its high growth fraction. Experience with chemotherapy has usually been in the setting of clinically extensive disease, with multiple organ involvement. Yet as single drugs, cyclophospamide (CTX), methotrexate (MTX), and adriamycin (ADR) have demonstrated objective response rates in the range of 33–46%.

Chemotherapy has a measurable effect on survival in extensive disease, as demonstrated by the controlled studies of the Veterans Administration Lung Study Group (VALSG) who found that CTX-treated patients survived a median of 17 weeks from the start of treatment, as compared to 7 weeks for a placebo-treated control $(p < 0.0005)$. More recently, uncontrolled studies and comparative studies of drugs alone or in combination have confirmed this, with a suggestion of superior survival for patients receiving combinations in most series. Median survivals in the range of 27 to 35 weeks are representative of results using the combination drug approach.

In spite of the responsiveness of systemic USC carcinoma to combination chemotherapy, the brain appears to act as a pharmacologic sanctuary from the effects of most drugs, and CNS relapse is a common problem in the presence of well-controlled disease elsewhere. The overall frequency of brain metastases in this tumor type has been reported at 30·5%; although 80% of brain metastases in this series were diagnosed ante-mortem, nearly half the patients died as a direct result. In other words, once CNS relapse occurs, radiotherapy and steroid management yield poor results.

Prognostic variables, which are important to keep in mind when discussing the chemotherapy of lung cancer include, besides histological type, performance status, extent of disease and prior therapy. Recent studies have confirmed the earlier reports of Karnofsky and others, that the performance status represents perhaps the single most important prognostic variable for survival and chemotherapy responsiveness in bronchogenic carcinoma. All comparative studies should stratify for this variable and it is difficult to assess the meaning of survival in any study without knowing the performance status of the patients entered.

Objective response is difficult to measure in lung cancer, since many cases do not present radiographic lesions which can be clearly measured by calipers in two dimensions; because of this the literature is replete with studies of the same drugs or regimens giving widely differing response rates. Some groups choose only to look at the survival as their therapeutic study end-point because of this measurement problem. The situation is further complicated by the fact that in many studies objective response does not correlate with any survival benefit. One explanation for this could be that the shrinkage observed in the X-ray may represent diminished pneumonitis and atelectasis due to relief of bronchial obstruction, rather than a major degree of neoplastic cell kill.

It is not uncommon in earlier studies to see objective response rates of 20–30% for single agents such as Cyclophosphamide, Nitrogen Mustard and Methotrexate reported. More recent studies have indicated that the true response rate for these agents as well as most others, is significantly less and is under 10% in many cases. There is no evidence that any single agent in the treatment of lung cancer causes a meaningful survival gain in any series of patients (Wasserman et al., 1975; Selawry and Hansen, 1973; Selawry, 1973).

E. *Malignant Melanoma*

5-(3,3-Dimethyl-1-triazeno)-imadazole-4-carboxamide (DTIC) has been the most extensively studied single agent in malignant melanoma.

The overall response rate for this drug is 25% in over 800 cases recently reviewed with great consistency in many large series.

Complete response rates of 5–6% have been consistently observed in each of the large studies with an overall remission rate of 5%.

In the reports on all major series, responders have lived longer than non-responders, as might be expected.

In view of the propensity of malignant melanoma to metastasise to the brain, the nitrosourea class of anti-tumor compounds are of particular interest because of their relatively high lipid solubility and ability to cross the blood-brain barrier.

The first generation nitrosourea, BCNU, has undergone extensive clinical trials. Published data, relating only to objective response rate, are currently available for 122 patients showing a response rate of 13%.

CCNU (1-(2-chloroethyl)-3-cyclohexyl-1-nitrosourea), the first oral congener of BCNU, has an objective response rate of 13% in 133 patients with disseminated maligant melanoma.

Methyl-CCNU, which is the newest nitrosourea to enter clinical trials, has shown response rates in excess of 20% and appears to be clinically as effective as DTIC.

A variety of other single agents have been investigated in this disease with only a few responses. Bleomycin, a drug that localizes in the skin, has thus far been totally inactive. Adriamycin has a broad spectrum of activity in solid tumors, but has shown no activity in melanoma. Initial reports of activity for pregnentrione and trimethylcolchicinic acid were never substantiated in larger studies.

While combination chemotherapy has been extensively investigated, no regimen is clearly superior to single agents and this approach cannot be recommended.

Malignant melanoma is a complex disease in which not only the clinical stage, but also the level of invasion of the primary lesion, and possibly patient immunocompetence, strongly affect prognosis. The vast majority of the patients die from disseminated disease, which at presentation is already beyond the scope of the primary local treatment modality. Chemotherapy is the only systemic modality possessing a well-documented potential for tumor cell kill in advanced disease. Immunotherapy, although less well documented, may be capable of controlling subclinical disease, occasionally widespread subcutaneous disease, and possibly enhancing the effect of chemotherapy in advanced disease. The integration of these modalites in a multi-faceted adjuvant attack on disease in high-risk patients might lead to greater control or actual eradication of the sub-clinical disease to which these patients ultimately succumb (Comis and Carter, S. K., 1974c).

F. *Ovary*

Alkylating agents have been utilized more extensively in patients with advanced ovarian cancer than any other class of chemotherapeutic agents. The initial response rates for various drugs in this class are around 35–65%, with 5–15% of all treated patients continuing to respond two years after initiation of therapy.

Available information does not suggest particular advantages for one alkylating agent over another and all appear to have approximately equal activity. Furthermore, no particular dose or schedule has been shown to be superior as similar response rates have been achieved with daily oral doses, oral loading doses, and intermittent intravenous doses.

Intraperitoneal administration of alkylating agents has been frequently advocated, although there is little evidence that it is effective or even equivalent to the effect of the same agent administered systemically. Generally the intraperitoneal use of alkylating agents has been reported to be less effective than the intravenous use of the same drug and dosage.

Patients with ovarian carcinoma who have received previous therapy will be less responsive to subsequent treatment with alkylating agents. In a large series where cyclophosphamide was used, there was a 75% response rate in previously untreated patients but only a 42% response rate in those relapsing after, or refractory to radiotherapy.

Alkylating agent chemotherapy as an adjuvant to initial surgery or radiotherapy in localized disease is currently of considerable interest, although few such studies have been published. At this time one cannot make definitive conclusions but further exploration of adjuvant chemotherapy in Stage 1 disease is warranted and is in progress in several randomized clinical trials.

Drugs other than the alkylating agents have been investigated much less completely in ovarian carcinoma. Before non-alkylating agents have been utilized, the patients have often failed therapy with alkylating agents, as well as radiation therapy and might therefore be expected to respond poorly to subsequent chemotherapy.

The antimetabolite 5-fluorouracil (5-FU) has been the most extensively studied of the non-alkylating agents and, regardless of schedule, appears to have a response rate of approximately 32%. Because of the extensive prior chemotherapy and/or radiotherapy that many of the patients received, direct comparison of 5-FU activity to that of the alkylating agents is not possible from the retrospective data.

Hexamethylmelamine has shown consistent activity in several trials against ovarian cancer. The drug is a derivative of the alkylating agent triethylenemelamine but is not felt to act primarily as an alkylating agent and has dose-limiting gastro-intestinal and neuro-toxicity, rather than bone marrow suppression. Furthermore, it is now clear that the drug is active in some patients with ovarian carcinoma who have become refractory to conventional alkylating agents.

A prospective randomized clinical trial comparing chemotherapy with 5-FU, hexamethylmelamine or melphalan in previously untreated patients with stage III and IV ovarian carcinoma, indicates an overall complete and partial response rate of 34% for melphalan, 53% for hexamethylmelamine, and 17% for 5-FU. If the high response rate to hexamethylmelamine continues to be documented in other trials, and if the durations of such responses are equivalent to those achieved with alkylating agents, hexamethylmelamine will be one of the most active single agents in the treatment of ovarian carcinoma.

The only anti-tumor antibiotic which has been studied in any detail is adriamycin. In a number of studies it is active as a single agent in both previously untreated patients and in those who have failed to respond to alkylating agent therapy. The overall response rate collected from the literature is 33%.

Because so few patients have been treated with the wide variety of non-alkylating agents mentioned above and because of the great variability of prior therapy and extent of disease, it is difficult to provide information on the median duration of response or the median survival of those patients so treated. This information is vital to properly assess the role of these agents *vis-à-vis* the alkylating agents. Only when definitive information is available on the extent of activity of these agents with different mechanisms of action and types of toxicity, will the rational design of combination chemotherapy regimens be possible.

Only a small number of studies of combination chemotherapy have been published in which more than a few patients with ovarian carcinoma were included. There are no data to support routine use of any combination at this time.

Radiotherapy and chemotherapy have been frequently combined in the management of patients with advanced disease. Unfortunately, the patients in many of these studies have represented a bewildering assortment of differing stages, histological types, grades, and previously treated patients who received chemotherapy before, after, or during radiotherapy either in sequence or because of failure of primary radiotherapeutic management. In some studies, patients failed radiotherapy either in sequence or because of failure of primary radiotherapeutic management. In some studies, patients failing radiotherapy were dropped from study before receiving chemotherapy and in others 5-year survivals with radiotherapy alone were calculated without consideration of whether subsequent chemotherapy was administered. It is difficult, if not impossible, to evaluate such studies and assess the true contribution of the combined modality approach to the management of advanced ovarian carcinoma. Only prospective studies of well-staged patients systematically given simultaneous or closely sequential radiotherapy and chemotherapy, would demonstrate synergistic effects of the two modalities if such a synergy exists (DeVita et al., in press; Young et al., 1974).

G. Head and Neck

Methotrexate has been the most extensively studied drug in head and neck cancer. It has been administered either by continuous intra-arterial (IA) infusion, or by systemic routes (IV or PO) with or without leucovorin "rescue". All of these approaches have shown significant anti-tumor activity, but unfortunately the available data do not permit a definitive choice of an optimum approach.

A review of the literature shows a 53% response rate in cases treated by IA methotrexate: this compares to an overall 40% response rate for systemic methotrexate on a variety of schedules. The responsiveness to IA infusion is not that impressive when one considers that the patients elected for this mode of therapy undoubtedly constituted a group having more localized disease.

When the toxicity of IA infusion is examined, the justification for this approach becomes questionable. In view of the fact that infusion has not given results superior to systemic use of the drug, further study of this approach does not appear to be indicated.

Systemic methotrexate has been given predominately by either an intermittent weekly or bi-weekly IV injection, or as monthly courses of a five-dose programme of oral or IV drug administration. The data for the weekly or bi-weekly approach show that 50% of the patients achieve 50% reduction in tumor size, as compared to 29% of those on monthly courses. This apparently indicates superiority for weekly or bi-weekly methotrexate administration. Other schedules that have shown activity include IV injection every two weeks and 1 to 3 mg/kg over 24 hours by continuous infusion, plus leucovorin in some cases.

The experimental basis of the methotrexate-calcium leucovorin approach derives from studies of Goldin showing that leucovorin, given 12 to 24 hours after methotrexate, improves the therapeutic index of the drug in mice bearing the L1210 leukaemia. Studies in head and neck cancer have produced $> 50\%$ reduction of tumor size in 43% of patients which again does not appear superior to results achieved with systemic methotrexate alone. In one recent study, patients were randomized to either methotrexate alone (80 to 110 mg/m^2) as a 30-hour infusion or over 36 to 42 hours (240 to 1080 mg/m^2) with leucovorin rescue. In both cases the infusions were administered every two weeks. The response rate among patients receiving methotrexate alone was 44% while it was 52% in the combined group, which indicates no meaningful difference.

Bleomycin, has shown activity against squamous cell carcinoma of the head and neck. There is an overall response rate of 31%. However, if only responses of $> 50\%$ tumor shrinkage are accepted this rate falls to only 15% and the mean duration of remission is quite short. Clearly, bleomycin is inferior to methotrexate as a single agent but its lack of bone-marrow toxicity makes it a prime candidate for combination regimens.

There are also indications of activity of cyclophosphamide, 5-FU, and hydroxyurea but the data are so limited when various tumor sites are considered that no definitive statement can be made.

Combination regimens have only been investigated to a limited extent and usually have not been designed specifically for head and neck cancer. The results with single agents do provide a basis for combination studies by demonstrating that head and neck cancer is responsive to drugs with differing mechanisms of action and without completely overlapping toxicities.

It is quite apparent that there has not yet been a clear delineation of the role of chemotherapy in combination with surgery and radio-therapy in the treatment of early head and neck cancer. There is evidence suggesting that therapeutic enhancement by chemotherapy can be obtained in tumors at specific sites, notably the oral cavity and maxillary sinuses. However, there has been no demonstration that IA perfusion affords better results than those obtained by systemic administration of the same drug. Similarly, no judgments can be made of the relative efficacy of one drug over another as an adjuvant to surgery and radiotherapy (Bertino *et al.*, 1973; Goldsmith and Carter, S. K., 1975).

H. *CNS Tumors*

Evaluation of objective response to chemotherapy in brain-tumor patients is exceedingly difficult when survival statistics are not available. So-called objective measurements of tumor size as determined by brain scan or angiogram are notoriously inaccurate. The brain scan cannot distinguish tumor from surrounding cerebral edema, nor viable from necrotic tumor. It has been shown that the brain scan did not agree with the clinical assessment of patient improvement or deterioration in 27% of 150 sequential scans. There was positive correlation of parallel carotid arteiograms in only 42% of cases. This, then, would leave the objective evaluation of response mainly to the clinical assessment of the patient. Given the vagaries of cerebral edema, especially where the use of steroids is uncontrolled, one must be skeptical to the critical evaluation of an objective response.

The nitrosoureas are probably the only drugs that are genuinely active in this disease. BCNU produces a response rate of 46% with a definitive prolongation of survival over no therapy following surgery. When combined with radiotherapy, the survival exceeds that of either modality alone. Fewer patients have been studied with CCNU and MeCCNU, but the response rates are roughly similar. These drugs are highly lipid-soluble, which explain their activity in glioblastoma. Assuming this is the case, further attention should be directed to cytotoxic drugs possessing this physical property.

In the miscellaneous class of antitumor agents, three drugs are interesting. Procarbazine has CNS toxicity and may also exert a cytotoxic effect but the data, although promising, are as yet not sufficient for a definitive statement. VM-26 is active against intracerebral L1210 leukaemia and preliminary studies indicate it may be an active agent against glioblastoma (Broder and Rall, 1972; Goldsmith and Carter, S. K., 1973; Wilson and Levin, 1975).

I. *Testicular Tumors*

The chemotherapy of testicular neoplasms has a long history of success, from the standpoint that these tumors have been shown to be responsive to a wide range of anti-cancer drugs. Active drugs include vinblastine (52%), actinomycin D (52%), mithramycin (36%), bleomycin (42%), melphalan (57%) and adriamycin (20%).

It is interesting to note that the concept of combining anti-tumor drugs, which has proven so valuable in the haematologic malignancies, had one of its first applications more than a decade ago in testicular tumors. In 1960, Li *et al.* published the first account of treatment with a three-drug combination in metastatic testicular cancer. This report and a subsequent one employed a regimen of chlorambucil, methotrexate and actinomycin D (Carter, S. K. and Wasserman, 1975).

Among 28 patients treated, there were 10 complete and 4 partial remissions; at least 1 of the complete responses occurred in a patient with choriocarcinoma.

A summary of extensive studies with this combination in a variety of centres has shown an overall response rate of 45% in 236 patients with 12% obtaining a complete response.

The discovery of bleomycin as an active agent in testicular carcinoma has had a major impact on the combination regimens currently utilized. At the M. D. Anderson Hospital a study combining bleomycin with vinblastine for the therapy of testicular tumours was undertaken and fifty patients were treated by this induction scheme. Sixteen patients achieved CR (32%) with this regimen and 15 were free of disease after two years. Twenty-two other patients experienced partial remission (50% reduction in maximum tumor diameter) with a median survival of 32 weeks.

In a modified approach to this regimen the complete response rate is 47% with an overall response of 75%. Mean survival of complete responders is 34 + weeks with none dead. It appears that the complete response rate is superior to intermittent bleomycin + vinblastine.

At the Memorial Sloan-Kettering Cancer Center, daily doses of a 3-drug combination of bleomycin, actinomycin D and vinblastine have been tried in testicular cancer. Twenty-one patients were treated and 16 were evaluable; of these, 8 showed objective responses lasting 1–5 months.

I. Actinomycin D 0·5 mg/d on days 3–7, 12–16, 21–25
   Chlorambucil 10 mg/d p.o. × 16–25 days
   Methotrexate 5 mg/d p.o. × 16–25 days

II. Vinblastine
    Bleomycin 0·4 mg/kg i.v. in 2 fractions (day 1 & 2)
    15 mg i.m. twice weekly × 10

III. VAB-I
     Vinblastine 0·025–0·05 mg/kg i.v. days 1, 2, 3
     Actinomycin D 0·0075–0·015 mg/kg repeated in 2–3
     Bleomycin 0·4 mg/kg doses in 7–14 days as toxicity permits

IV. VAB-II
    Change Bleomycin to 0·5 mg/kg/d × 7 by continuous infusion
    Add Cis-platinum diamminedichloride 1 mg/kg i.v. on day 7

V. Actinomycin D   0·4 mg/m² i.v. days 1–5
   Vincristine   1 mg/m² i.v. days 1 & 8
   Bleomycin   15 mg/m² i.v. days 1, 8, 15

FIG. 7. Commonly utilized combinations in testicular cancer

A modification of this approach involved bleomycin by continuous IV infusion combined with cis-platinum diammine dichloride. Sixteen previously treated patients with germ-cell tumors have been treated with this regimen. All were resistant to conventional weekly IV bleomycin and had been exposed to vinblastine and actinomycin D. Eleven of the patients had partial responses lasting 2–7 + months with one additional patient having a minor response (< 50% > 1 month).

It is clear that with the use of aggressive combination chemotherapy a certain number of patients can achieve long-term disease free control. These regimens should not be attempted by inexperienced clinicians or in hospitals without adequate supportive care facilities. Since this is a rare tumor, which strikes man in the prime of life, every effort should be made to get patients to an adequate treatment facility, since cure is a distinct possibility with proper therapy (Samuels, 1975; Silvay et al., 1973; Cvitkovic et al., 1975; Blom and Brodovsky, 1975)

References

Aur, R., Simone, J. and Hustu, O. (1971). Central nervous system therapy and combination chemotherapy of childhood lymphocytic leukemia. Blood, 37, 272–281.

Baker, L. H. Matter, R., Talley, R. (1975). 5-FU vs. 5-FU and MeCCNU in gastrointestinal cancer. A phase II study of the Southwest Oncology Group. Proc. Am. Assoc. Cancer Res. 16, 229.

Bertino, R. J., Mosher, M. B. and DeConti, R. C. (1973). Chemotherapy of cancer of the head and neck. Cancer, 31, 1141–1149.

Blom, J. and Brodovsky, H. S. (1975). Comparison of the treatment of metastatic testicular tumors with actinomycin D or actinomycin D, bleomycin and vincristine. Proc. Am. Assoc. Cancer Res. 16, 247.

Brewer, J. I., Dolkard, R. E., Torok, E. E. (1970) Gestational trophoblastic disease. In "Proceedings of the Sixth National Cancer Conference", pp. 387–395. Lippincott, Philadelphia.

Broder, L. E. and Rall, D. P. (1972). Chemotherapy of brain tumors. Prog. Exp. Tumor Res. 17, 373–379.

Broder, L. E. and Tormey, D. C. (1974). Combination chemotherapy of carcinoma of the breast. Cancer Treat. Rev. 1, 183–203.

Carter, S. K. (1972). Single and combination nonhormonal chemotherapy in breast cancer. Cancer, 30, 1543–1555.

Carter, S. K. (1974). The chemical therapy of breast cancer. Semin. Oncol. 1, 131–144.

Carter, S. K. (1975). Testicular neoplasms: prognostic factors and criteria of response. *In* "Cancer Therapy: Prognostic Factors and Criteria of Response" (M. Staquet, ed.), pp. 255–268. Raven Press, New York.

Carter, S. K. (1976). Large bowel cancer—the current status of treatment. *J. Natl. Cancer Inst.* **56**, 3–10.

Carter, S. K. and Livingston, R. (1973). Single agent therapy of Hodgkin's disease. *Arch. Intern. Med.* **131**, 377–387.

Carter, S. K. and Soper, W. T. (1974). Integration of chemotherapy into combined modality treatment of solid tumours. I. The overall strategy. *Cancer Treat. Rev.* **1**, 1–13.

Carter S. K. and Wasserman, T. H. (1975). The chemotherapy of urologic cancer. *Cancer*, **36**, 729–747.

Comis, R. L. and Carter, S. K. (1974a). Integration of chemotherapy into a combined modality treatment of solid tumors. III. Gastric cancer. *Cancer Treat. Rev.* **1**, 221–238.

Comis, R. L. and Carter, S. K. (1974b). A review of chemotherapy in gastric cancer. *Cancer*, **34**, 1576–1586.

Comis, R. K. and Carter, S. K. (1974c). Integration of chemotherapy into combined modality treatment of solid tumors. IV. Malignant melanoma. *Cancer Treat. Rev.* **1**, 285–304.

Cortes, E. P., Holland, J. F., Wang. J. J. (1974). Amputation and adriamycin in primary osteosarcoma. *New Engl. J. Med.* **291**, 988.

Cvitkovic, E., Currie, V., Krakoff, I. H. (1975). Bleomycin infusion with cis-platinum diamminedichloride as secondary chemotherapy for germinal cell tumors. *Proc. Am. Assoc. Cancer Res.* **16**, 273.

DeVita, V. T., Serpick, A. A. and Carbone, P. P. (1970). Combination chemotherapy in the treatment of advanced Hodgkin's disease. *Ann. Intern. Med.* **73**, 881–895.

DeVita, V. T., Wasserman, T. H., Young. R. C. Perspectives on research in gynecologic oncology. *Cancer*. In press.

Ellsworth, R. M. (1968). Treatment of retinoblastoma. *Am. J. Opthalmol.* **66**, 49–51.

Farber, S. (1966). Chemotherapy in the treatment of leukemia and Wilms' tumor. *J.A.M.A.* **198**, 826–836.

Fisher, B., Carbone, P., Economou, E. (1975). L-Phenylalanine mustard (L-PAM) in the management of primary breast cancer: a report of early findings. *New Engl. J. Med.* **292**, 117–122.

Goldsmith, M. A. and Carter, S. K. (1973). Clioblastoma multiforme: a review of therapy. *Cancer Treat. Rev.* **1**, 153–165.

Goldsmith, M. A. and Carter, S. K. (1975). Integration of chemotherapy into combined modality treatment of solid tumors. V. Squamous cell carcinoma of the head and neck. *Cancer Treat. Rev.* **2**, 137–158.

Henderson, E. S. (1969). Treatment of acute leukemia. *Semin. Hematol.* **6**, 271–319.

Holland, J. F. and Hreshchyshyn, M. M. (eds) (1967). "Choriocarcinoma". Union Internationale Contre le Cancer Monograph Series, Vol. 3. Springer-Verlag, Heidelberg.

Holland, J. F. and Glidewell, O. (1970). Complementary chemotherapy in acute leukemia. *Recent Results Cancer Res.* **30**, 95–108.

Holland, J. F., Hreshchysyn, M. M. and Glidewell, O. (1971). Controlled clinical trials of methotrexate in treatment and prophylaxis of trophoblastic disease. *In* "Oncology" (R. L. Clark, R. W. Cumley and J. E. McKay, eds), pp. 220–227, Vol. IV. Year Book Medical Publishers, Chicago.

Hustu, H. O., Holten, C., James, P. (1968). Treatment of Ewing's sarcoma with concurrent radiotherapy and chemotherapy. *J. Pediatr.* **73**, 249–251.

Jaffe, N., Frei, E., Traggis, D. (1974) Adjuvant methotrexate and citrovorum factor treatment of osteogenic sarcoma. *New Engl. J. Med.* **291**, 994–997.

Mackenzie, A. R. (1966). Chemotherapy of metastatic testis cancer: results in 154 patients. *Cancer*, **19**, 1369–1376.

Moertel, C. G. (1975). Clinical management of advanced gastrointestinal cancer. *Cancer*, **36**, 675–682.

Moertel, C. G., Schutt, A. J., Hahn, R. G. (1975). Therapy of advanced colorectal cancer with a combination of 5-fluorouracil, methyl-1-3-cis (2-chloroethyl)-1-nitrosourea, and vincristine. *J. Natl. Cancer Inst.* **54**, 69–71.

Peters, M. V. (1971). Historical perspectives in Hodgkin's disease. *In* "Oncology" (R. L. Clark, R. W. Cumley, and J. E. McKay, eds), Vol. IV, pp. 483–493. Year Book Medical Publishers, Chicago.

Pratt, C. B., Hustu, H. O., Fleming, I. P. (1972). Coordinated treatment of childhood rhabdomyosarcoma with surgery, radiotherapy and combination chemotherapy. *Cancer Res.* **32**, 606–610.

Samuels, M. L. (1975). Continuous intravenous bleomycin therapy with vinblastine in testicular and extragonadal germinal tumors. *Proc. Am. Assoc. Cancer Res.* **16**, 112.

Selawry, O. S. (1973). Monochemotherapy of bronchogenic carcinoma with special reference to cell type. *Cancer Chemother. Rep.* **4**, 177–188.

Selawry, O. S. and Hansen, H. H. (1973). Lung cancer. *In* "Cancer Medicine" (J. F. Holland and E. Frei, eds), pp. 1473–1518. Lea & Febiger, Philadelphia.

Silvay, O., Yagoda, A., Wittes, R. (1973). Treatment of germ cell carcinomas with a combination of actinomycin D, vinblastine, and bleomycine. *Proc. Am. Assoc. Cancer Res.* **14**, 68.

Skipper, H. E., Schabel, F. M. and Wilcox, W. S. (1964). Experimental evaluation of potential anticancer agents XIII. On the criteria and kinetics associated with "Curability" of experimental leukemia. *Cancer Chemother. Rep.* **35**, 1–111.

Sullivan, M. P. and Sutow, W. W. (1969). Successful therapy for Wilms' tumor. *Tex. Med.* **65**, 46–51.

Sutow, W. W., Gehan, E. A., Heyn, R. M. (1970). Comparison of survival curves 1956 versus 1962, in children with Wilms' tumor and neuroblastoma. *Pediatrics*, **45**, 800–811.

Sutow, W. W., Sullivan, M. P., Fernbach, D. J. (1975). Adjuvant chemotherapy in primary treatment of osteogenic sarcoma. *Cancer*, **36**, 1598–1602.

Wasserman, T. H., Comis, R. L., Goldsmith, M. (1975). Tabular analysis of the clinical chemotherapy of solid tumors. *Cancer Chemother. Rep.* **6**, 399–419.

Wilbur, J., Sutow, W., Sullivan, M. L. (1971). Successful treatment of rhabdomyosarcoma with combination chemotherapy and radiotherapy. *In* "Proceedings of the American Society of Clinical Oncology". Chicago.

Wilson, C. B. and Levin, V. A. (1975). Brain tumors. *In* "Clinical Cancer Chemotherapy" (E. M. Greenspan, ed.), Chapter 16, pp. 297–312. Raven Press, New York.

Young, R. C., Hubbard, S. P. and DeVita, V. T. (1974). The chemotherapy of ovarian carcinoma. *Cancer Treat. Rev.* **1**, 99–110.

Index